MRCOG Part 2

Essential EMQs

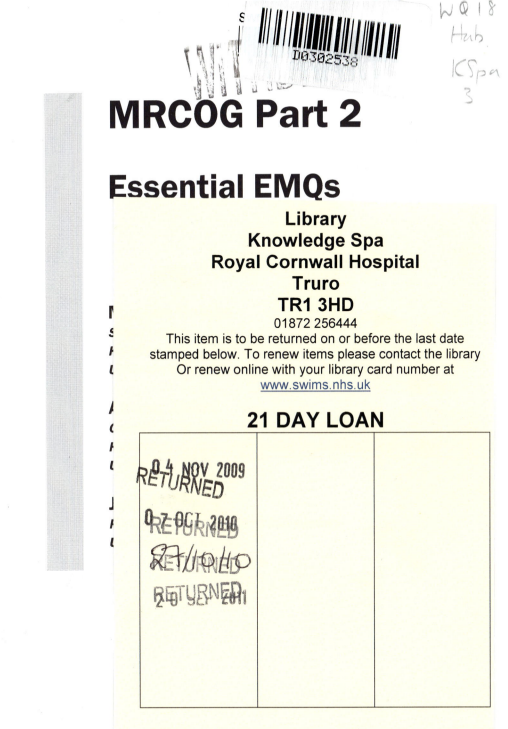

Radcliffe Publishing

Oxford ● New York

Radcliffe Publishing Ltd
18 Marcham Road
Abingdon
Oxon OX14 1AA
United Kingdom

www.radcliffe-oxford.com
Electronic catalogue and worldwide online ordering facility.

New research and clinical experience can result in changes in treatment and drug therapy. Readers of this book should therefore check the most recent product information on any drug they may prescribe to ensure they are complying with the manufacturer's recommendations concerning dosage, the method and duration of administration, and contraindications. Neither the publisher nor the authors accept liability for any injury or damage arising from this publication.

British Library Cataloguing in Publication Data

A catalogue record for this book is available from the British Library.

ISBN-13 978 1 84619 032 2

Typeset by Advance Typesetting Ltd, Oxford
Printed and bound by TJI Digital, Padstow, Cornwall

Contents

Foreword

One of the highlights of any specialist medical professionals' life is success in their final examination, thereby giving them their final passage of entry into their chosen speciality. Professional examinations have evolved over the latter part of the 20th and beginning of the 21st Century, gradually becoming more relevant to clinical practice, testing competences and attitudes directly relevant to the provision of high-quality clinical care. A recent example of these developments has been the introduction of EMQs. The Royal College of Obstetricians and Gynaecologists, consistent with its history of being at the forefront of new developments in medical education and training, has included EMQs in its examinations.

My colleagues in Leicester have found the energy and commitment to make their own contributions to this development. This book will provide excellent preparation for those about to take the MRCOG Examination, but will also be of use to more junior colleagues as they develop skills in their speciality.

I am sure you will find it a most helpful book in your professional journey.

Professor David J Taylor MD, FRCOG
Professor of Obstetrics and Gynaecology and Vice Dean
Leicester Medical School, University of Leicester
June 2007

Preface

In 2006, the Royal College of Obstetricians and Gynaecologists successfully introduced extended matching questions (EMQs) into the Part 2 membership examination, and familiarity with this question format has become a necessity for MRCOG candidates. The number of published revision aids including this question format in postgraduate obstetrics and gynaecology remains limited. With this book we wanted to produce a comprehensive selection of EMQs, covering broad areas relevant to the speciality, which would be useful to those preparing for postgraduate examinations at Part 2 MRCOG level or equivalent. This work brought together two authors with MRCOG examination committee experience, namely Justin Konje (Part 2) and Marwan Habiba (Part 1), and Andrea Akkad's special interest in medical education and her experience in creating an undergraduate EMQ database for students at the University of Leicester, where the authors studied and continue to teach.

By its very nature, this book is not designed as a source book, and the candidate is advised to refer to the RCOG Part 2 membership examination syllabus for a comprehensive coverage of the content. We have included a list of text- and reference books recommended for revision for postgraduate examinations in obstetrics and gynaecology, and further information on relevant literature can be accessed on the RCOG website (www.rcog.org.uk).

We hope that you will find this book proves helpful as a study guide, particularly for those preparing for the MRCOG Part 2 or equivalent postgraduate examinations.

Marwan Habiba
Andrea Akkad
Justin Konje
June 2007

About the authors

Mr Marwan Habiba MSc PhD FRCOG is a senior lecturer and honorary consultant in obstetrics and gynaecology at the University of Leicester. He obtained a PhD in medicine on 'Endometrial Responses to Hormone Replacement Therapy' (1998) and a PhD in philosophy on 'Health Screening: a libertarian perspective' (2000). Mr Habiba pursues his research interest in the endometrium, healthcare delivery and ethics, and he leads a workshop on medical ethics for Leicester medical students. He currently serves on the MRCOG Part 1 Examination Committee.

Dr Andrea Akkad MD MRCOG is a consultant/lead for undergraduate education in obstetrics and gynaecology and honorary senior lecturer in medical and social care education at the University of Leicester and the University Hospitals of Leicester NHS Trust. Her main areas of interest in medical education are assessment and standard setting. She is a keen question writer, and has recently led the successful conversion of the written undergraduate O&G exams in Leicester to an EMQ-based assessment format.

Professor Justin Konje MD FMCOG (Nig) MRCOG holds a chair in obstetrics and gynaecology at the University of Leicester. His clinical and research interests include fetal growth disorders, recurrent miscarriage and endometriosis. Throughout his career Professor Konje has had a keen interest in medical education, and has contributed substantially to undergraduate obstetrics and gynaecology in Leicester. He currently serves on the MRCOG Part 2 Examination Committee.

Introduction

The Part 2 MRCOG examination

Preparing for the Part 2 MRCOG examination remains a daunting and complex task, particularly as learning and revision often need to fit around clinical commitments. Much has been written about how to prepare for and pass exams, yet it remains surprising how often well-read candidates provide unsatisfactory answers in areas which they 'know' well. Clearly, a sound understanding of the topic area is essential, but deeper knowledge also increases uncertainty, and the vast developments in the field mean that proficiency in all areas is next to impossible. Thus a critical point for postgraduate candidates, who more often than not will prepare for the examination in isolation, is to develop a real understanding of what the examination is meant to assess.

The format of the examination itself has passed through several evolutionary stages. Long essays were supplanted by short essays, and most candidates are now familiar with multiple-choice questions (MCQs). So why is the Royal College of Obstetricians and Gynaecologists keen to introduce yet another format?

Essay writing requires particular linguistic skills and thus may disadvantage some, who may otherwise achieve the required standard without much difficulty. MCQs are good at assessing factual recall, but EMQs have the added advantage of being able to assess 'interpretational' skill and judgement, with less cueing and reliance on elimination of obviously incorrect answers. Besides, a good EMQ can enact a credible clinical scenario and thus render the examination more 'clinically' relevant, a feature which ranks highly on the RCOG's priorities for the membership examination. On the other hand, EMQs can be time-consuming and difficult to set to the required standard, and may not be satisfactorily applicable across the syllabus. As such, it is very likely that MCQs will still feature in membership examinations for years to come, but

EMQs will form an increasingly important component of most postgraduate examinations, at least in the UK.

What is an EMQ?

The aim of this book is to introduce candidates to the EMQ format applied to postgraduate obstetrics and gynaecology. Well-constructed EMQs have a common structure and would usually include four components:

1 theme – the topic covered by the question, e.g. investigating abdominal pain in pregnancy; this may be explicitly stated in a heading or implied by the uniform question content
2 option list – a list of possible answers, e.g. a list of investigations you might consider performing when investigating abdominal pain in pregnancy
3 lead-in statement or instruction – directs the candidate to the specific task required, e.g. select the single most useful investigation from the option list
4 at least two item stems – ideally clinical vignettes or case histories, but can include short statements in some questions.

We have not specifically named the theme for each group of stems, but have left that for the candidate to deduce from the instruction, option list and case mix given under each heading – this is the style used in the MRCOG Part 2 examination.

The option list for EMQs should be homogeneous and plausible; it may consist of single words, short phrases, tabulated laboratory values or images. The most important feature of the EMQ format is that it requires the candidate to *interpret* the stem, and not simply to solve a puzzle by linking the stem to the most appropriate item on the option list. This means that, in some questions, a number of answers may sound plausible; however, the specific circumstances of the clinical scenario should direct the candidate to choose the most suitable answer.

When answering EMQs, it is not thought to be particularly useful to go through the option list in an effort to eliminate incorrect answers. Firstly, there may be a long list of answers, and secondly, you are often selecting a *best* answer amongst a number of possibles, rather than making a *true/false* judgement on each option. The stem will contain clues to direct you to the best answer, so read it very carefully.

The most useful approach to the EMQ is to read the instruction and the stem or vignette first, and then try to answer the question *before* looking at the option list; when you do then read the options, you will be less distracted by other answers on the list. If the answer you thought of does not appear on the list, read the stem again to make sure you haven't overlooked any important details.

Setting the standard

Although one should aim high, no candidate should expect to correctly answer 100% of the questions! A hotly debated question amongst candidates – especially those who may not be familiar with standard setting – is the examination pass mark. There is no fixed pass mark for the MRCOG examination; neither does the college predetermine the proportion of candidates who pass or fail. Instead, the pass mark is decided for each examination based on the difficulty of the particular paper.

Whilst EMQs may vary in style and complexity, the basic structure and the approach to answering them remain the same. With some practice, you should be able to successfully answer questions in EMQ format.

Reading list

Textbooks

Chamberlain G. *Turnbulls Obstetrics* (3e). Churchill Livingstone; 2001. ISBN: 0443063656.

Drife J, Magowan B. *Clinical Obstetrics and Gynaecology*. Saunders; 2004. ISBN: 00702017752.

Enkin M *et al*. *Guide to Effective Care in Pregnancy and Childbirth* (3e). Oxford University Press; 2000. ISBN: 019263173X.

Greer I, Cameron J, Kitchener H, Prentice A. *Colour Atlas and Text of Obstetrics and Gynaecology*. Mosby; 2000. ISBN: 0723424357.

James DK, Steer PJ, Weiner CP, Gonik B. *High-Risk Pregnancies: management options*. WB Saunders; 2005. ISBN: 0721601324.

Luesley D, Baker P. *Obstetrics and Gynaecology: an evidence-based text for MRCOG*. Arnold; 2004. ISBN: 034808756.

Nelson-Piercy C. *Handbook of Obstetric Medicine*. Taylor and Francis; 2006. ISBN: 1841845809.

Shaw R, Soutter WP and Stanton SL. *Gynaecology* (3e). Churchill Livingstone; 2003. ISBN: 0443070296.

The following book series cover topics relevant to the MRCOG candidate:

Progress in Obstetrics and Gynaecology series, Elsevier.
Recent Advances in Obstetrics and Gynaecology series, RSM Press.
For the MRCOG and Beyond, RCOG Press.
Lewis G and CEMACH. *Why Mothers Die, 2000–2002. The Sixth Report of Confidential Enquiries into Maternal Deaths in the United Kingdom*. RCOG Press; 2004. ISBN: 190475208X.

Websites

Royal College of Obstetrics and Gynaecology (RCOG) guidelines: www.rcog.org.uk/index.asp?PageID=8
National Institute for Health and Clinical Excellence (NICE) guidelines: www.nice.org.uk/guidance/topic/gynaecology

Cochrane Database of Pregnancy and Childbirth: www.cochrane.org/
   reviews/en/topics/87.html
Scottish Intercollegiate Guidelines Network (SIGN) guidelines: www.
   sign.ac.uk/guidelines/published/#Obstetrics
Prodigy Clinical Knowledge Summaries: www.prodigy.nhs.uk/guidance/
   by_clinical_specialty/womens_health

Abbreviations

ABPM	ambulatory blood pressure monitoring
AC	abdominal circumference
ACTH	adrenocorticotropic hormone
AFI	amniotic fluid index
ALT	alanine transferase
ARM	artificial rupture of membranes
ASD	atrial septum defect
BMI	body mass index
BP	blood pressure
BSO	bilateral salpingo-oophorectomy
CAH	congenital adrenal hyperplasia
CIN	cervical intraepithelial neoplasia
COCP	combined oral contraceptive pill
CRH	corticotrophin-releasing hormone
CTG	cardiotocography
CXR	chest x-ray
DHEAS	dehydroepiandrosterone sulfate
DNA	deoxyribonucleic acid
DOA	direct occipitoanterior
DOP	direct occipito-posterior
DVT	deep vein thrombosis
ECG	electrocardiogram
FAI	free androgen index
FBC	full blood count
FBS	fetal blood sample
FSH	follicle-stimulating hormone
GDM	gestational diabetes mellitus
GnRH	gonadotrophin-releasing hormone
GP	general practitioner
GTT	glucose tolerance test
Hb	haemoglobin
HC	head circumference
HCG	human chorionic gonadotrophin
HIV	human immunodeficiency virus

HSG	hysterosalpingogram
ICSI	intracytoplasmatic sperm injection
IDDM	insulin-dependent diabetes mellitus
IM	intramuscular
INR	international normalised ratio
IOL	induction of labour
ITP	immune thrombocytopaenic purpura
IUCD	intrauterine contraceptive device
IUGR	intrauterine growth restriction
IUI	intrauterine insemination
IUS	intrauterine system
IVF	*in vitro* fertilisation
LH	luteinising hormone
LMP	last menstrual period
LNG	levonorgestrel
LOA	left occipitoanterior
MEA	microwave endometrial ablation
MSU	midstream specimen of urine
NIDDM	non-insulin-dependent diabetes mellitus
NTD	neural tube defect
NVD	normal vaginal delivery
OAB	overactive bladder
OP	occipitoposterior
PCOS	polycystic ovary syndrome
PID	pelvic inflammatory disease
POD	pouch of Douglas
POP	progestogen-only pill
RBBB	right bundle branch block
RNA	ribonucleic acid
ROP	right occipito-posterior
RPOC	retained products of conception
SC	subcutaneous
SNRI	serotonin and noradrenaline reuptake inhibitor
SSRI	selective serotonin reuptake inhibitor
TAH	total abdominal hysterectomy
TOP	termination of pregnancy
TSH	thyroid-stimulating hormone
TVT	transvaginal tape

USI	urodynamic stress incontinence
USS	ultrasound scan
UTI	urinary tract infection
VMA	vanillylmandelic acid
VSD	ventricular septum defect
WBC	white blood cell count

QUESTIONS

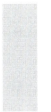

Applied basic sciences

Q1

Options:

A Müllerian agenesis
B Incomplete division of metanephric diverticulum
C Absent fusion of paramesonephric ducts
D Incomplete lateral fusion/septum resorption
E Right-sided Müllerian duct hypoplasia
F Incomplete vertical fusion of sinovaginal bulb with Müllerian system
G Absent mesonephric ducts
H Absence of Müllerian-inhibiting substance
I Incomplete fusion of paramesonephric ducts
J Agenesis of Wolffian ducts
K Left-sided Müllerian duct hypoplasia

Lead-in:

For each of the following presentations of genital tract mal-development, please select *the most likely embryological mechanism* from the option list. Each option may be used once, more than once, or not at all.

Q1 A 19-year-old woman is referred to a gynaecology clinic because of absent menstruation. Her thelarche and pubarche are both Tanner stage 5. Abdominal examination is unremarkable, and she appears to have normal external genitalia. An ultrasound scan reports normal ovaries, but insufficient bladder filling precludes any comment on size or shape of the uterus.

Q2 A 33-year-old woman undergoes a Caesarean section for a breech presentation at term. At Caesarean section the obstetrician can only identify one Fallopian tube, which is situated in the midline due to extreme dextro-rotation of the uterus.

Q3 A 29-year-old woman presents in the gynaecology clinic with a six-year history of primary infertility. You make a clinical assessment in outpatients, and can ascertain that the patient's cervix is duplicated.

Q4 A 16-year-old girl presents in the paediatric gynaecology clinic with her mother because of recurrent lower abdominal pain. She has not yet started to menstruate. On examination her thelarche and pubarche are Tanner stage 4; on abdominal palpation she has a tender mass arising from the pelvis.

Q5 A 41-year-old woman undergoes a hysteroscopy because of recurrent vaginal bleeding. She has a single cervix and lower uterine cavity, but a uterine septum is visualised in the upper part of the uterus.

Q2

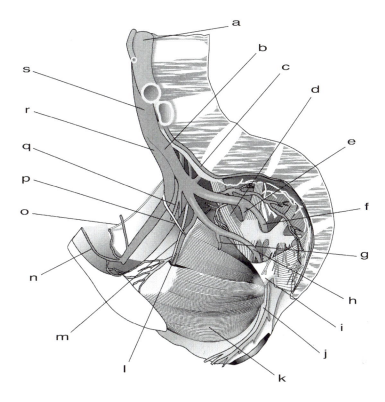

Lead-in:

For each clinical case of gynaecological surgery below, please select *the most relevant structure* from the diagram above. Each option may be used once, more than once, or not at all.

 A 30-year-old woman of Afro-Caribbean origin with multiple large uterine fibroids opts for a minimally invasive procedure. You arrange a consultation with an interventional radiologist.

A 79-year-old woman develops a vault prolapse following abdominal hysterectomy. You suggest a repair operation that can be performed vaginally.

 A 45-year-old woman undergoes an operation for cervical cancer. Postoperatively, she suffers with difficulty walking. She is noted to have external rotation of her right foot.

 A 76-year-old woman with a complete procidentia undergoes vaginal hysterectomy. Postoperatively, she is noted to be anuric, and does not respond to fluid challenge.

 A 35-year-old woman undergoes laparoscopic ablation to endometriosis. She develops a haematoma at the site of the ancillary port.

Q3
Options:

A   Femoral artery
B   Femoral nerve
C   Popliteal vein
D   Superior vesical artery
E   Ureter
F   Obturator nerve
G   External iliac vein
H   Pudendal nerve
I   Inferior vesical artery
J   Internal pudendal artery
K   Obturator artery
L   Genitofemoral nerve

Lead-in:

For each of the clinical presentations below, please select *the structure most likely to be of relevance*. Each option may be used once, more than once, or not at all.

Q11 A 28-year-old woman presents two days postpartum with severe pain in her left leg. On clinical examination there is redness and swelling of her left thigh.

Q12 A 24-year-old woman is admitted with left-sided colicky abdominal pain radiating to her left thigh. Diagnostic laparoscopy is negative.

Q13 A 38-year-old nulliparous woman presents with right-sided loin pain. Her periods are regular and not heavy. Further investigations reveal a cervical fibroid of 8 cm diameter.

Q14 A 24-year-old woman is noted to have a large vaginal haematoma following the administration of a nerve conduction block prior to ventouse delivery.

Q15 A 43-year-old woman undergoes an abdominal hysterectomy. Postoperatively, she complains of numbness and altered sensation in her right thigh and knee, and feels her knee 'giving way' whilst walking. She finds descending stairs particularly difficult. On examination she has weakness of hip flexion as well as knee extension.

Q4

Options:

A Diagonal conjugate
B Mentovertical circumference
C Suboccipitobregmatic circumference
D Bisacromial diameter

E   Occipitofrontal circumference
F   Submentobregmatic circumference
G   Obstetric conjugate
H   Pelvic axis
I   Curve of Carus
J   Suboccipitofrontal circumference
K   Biparietal diameter
L   True conjugate
M   Intertuberous diameter
N   Interspinous diameter

Lead-in:

For each of the following intrapartum scenarios, please select *the anatomical descriptor most relevant to adequate progress* from the option list. Each option may be used once, more than once, or not at all.

Q16 A 30-year-old primigravida is admitted to the labour ward in spontaneous labour at term. On vaginal examination her cervix is 5 cm dilated and the presenting part is at the level of the ischial spines +2. The sagittal and the lambda sutures can be readily palpated.

Q17 A 39-year-old grand multipara is admitted to the labour ward in spontaneous labour at term. Clinical examination reveals a pendulous abdomen. On vaginal examination the cervix is fully dilated and the presenting part is at the level of the ischial spines –2, with the sagittal suture palpated in left oblique diameter, and the coronal sutures are identified anteriorly.

Q18 A 27-year-old nulliparous woman of Indo-Asian origin, who has only recently arrived in the UK, presents to the labour ward in spontaneous labour, self-reportedly following an uncomplicated pregnancy. On clinical examination a term-size uterus is identified, with a long lie and a cephalic presentation; 5/5 of the head are palpable. On vaginal examination the cervix is 5 cm dilated and the membranes are intact and bulging. The presenting part is not reached, but the sacral promontory is readily palpable.

(Q19) A 23-year-old parous woman presents to the labour ward in early labour near term. Her membranes ruptured six hours after admission. Vaginal examination is carried out and the cervix is found to be fully dilated. The chin is palpated in the midline posteriorly.

(Q20) A 34-year-old primigravida presents to the labour ward in advanced spontaneous labour at 37 weeks' gestation. On vaginal examination her cervix is noted to be 7 cm dilated and the presenting part is at the level of the ischial spines +1. The sagittal suture is in the right oblique diameter, and both the anterior and posterior fontanelle can be readily palpated.

Q5

Options:

A   Mitochondrial inheritance
B   Trinucleotide repeat expansion
C   Genomic imprinting
D   Single gene mutation
E   Uniparental disomy
F   Non-disjunction
G   Somatic mosaicism
H   Missense mutation
I   Germline mosaicism
J   Confined placental mosaicism

Lead-in:

For each of the following scenarios, please select the *most relevant genetic mechanism* from the option list. Each option may be used once, more than once, or not at all.

(Q21) Patients with non-insulin-dependent diabetes mellitus (NIDDM) are more likely to have a mother who was diagnosed with NIDDM than a father. This suggests that this pattern of inheritance, which only occurs from mother to offspring, is responsible for a proportion of cases with NIDDM.

(Q22) One of the female X chromosomes is inactivated, resulting in dosage compensation so that the structural genes on the X chromosome are expressed at the same level in males and females.

(Q23) A 28-year-old woman presents for prenatal counselling. Her three-year-old child was noted to be hypotonic in the neonatal period, with poor feeding. At one year of age he was hyperphagic and consequently became obese. He has dysmorphic features, including a narrow bifrontal diameter and almond-shaped palpebral fissures; additionally he has cryptorchidism and a hypoplastic scrotum. On genetic work-up, an abnormality was detected involving band 15q11-q13.

(Q24) A 19-year-old woman with mild mental retardation presents for prenatal counselling. She is phenotypically normal. Results of genetic testing involving the FMR1 gene were consistent with the diagnosis of fragile X syndrome.

(Q25) A 25-year-old man presents for genetic counselling because of a family history of progressive chorea, dementia, rigidity and seizures. He tells you that several male members of his family have died at a young age.

Q6

Options:

A Background population risk
B 1:2
C 1:100
D 1:8
E 1:20
F 1:1000
G 1:4
H 1:10,000
I 1:200
J 1:500
K 1:250
L 3:4

Lead-in:

For each of the preconceptual counselling scenarios below, please select *the most appropriate risk of the fetus being affected.* Each option can be used once, more than once, or not at all.

 A 33-year-old African woman books at 12 weeks' gestation. Her antenatal blood tests reveal that she has a sickle cell trait. Her partner is also a carrier. She wishes to know the risk of sickle cell disease in the baby.

A 25-year-old woman had a baby with trisomy 21 in her previous pregnancy. There is no family history of aneuploidy or congenital malformations otherwise on her or her partner's side. She wishes to know the likely recurrence risk in her next pregnancy.

A dwarf couple attend for preconceptual counselling. The woman has achondroplasia, whilst the male partner has another form of non-lethal dwarfism; he was told his condition was non-hereditary. They would like to have a baby, and wish to know the likelihood of the baby having achondroplasia.

 A 41-year-old woman, who had a termination of pregnancy previously because of a fetal neural tube defect, finds herself pregnant. The pregnancy is unplanned, and she had not taken folate supplementation. She wishes to know the risk of her baby having a neural tube defect again.

Q30 A 22-year-old woman with congenital heart disease is pregnant for the first time. She herself had a large VSD repaired in infancy, and has had a functionally good result from surgery. She would like to know whether there is any risk of her baby having a cardiac defect.

Reproductive health

Q7

Options:

	First-year failure rate with ideal use	First-year failure rate with typical use
A	85%	85%
B	0.1%	3%
C	0.5%	33%
D	0.5%	3%
E	0.6%	0.8%
F	0.5%	0.5%
G	4%	20%
H	26%	40%
I	2%	15%
J	1%	20%
K	0.5%	10%
L	99%	95%

Lead-in:

For each contraceptive choice below, please select *the most appropriate efficacy figures* from the option list. Each option may be used once, more than once, or not at all.

(Q31) A 23-year-old woman using a second-generation COCP.

A 28-year-old woman using the levonorgestrel intrauterine system.

A 32-year-old woman who has been sterilised.

A 32-year-old woman using the withdrawal method.

A 26-year-old woman using male condoms.

Q8

Options:

A   1:5
B   28:10,000
C   1:10
D   1:1000
E   2:100
F   2:10,000
G   8:1000
H   5:100,000
I   4:100,000
J   4:1,000,000

Lead-in:

For each of the complications of family planning measures below, please select *the most appropriate incidence figure* from the option list. Each option may be used once, more than once, or not at all.

 A 26-year old, healthy nulliparous woman with a BMI of 27 uses a third-generation COCP. She is seeking advice about the risk of thromboembolism.

A 30-year-old parous woman is interested in starting the COCP for contraception and control of heavy periods. She has a family history of venous thromboembolism; although she herself has never had a thrombosis, she is known to have protein S deficiency.

 A 35-year-old parous woman wishes to have an IUCD inserted. She is enquiring about the risk of uterine perforation during insertion.

Q39 A 28-year-old, healthy nulliparous woman with a BMI of 27 uses a progestogen-only pill. She is seeking advice about the risk of thromboembolism.

Q40 A 19-year-old woman is scheduled to undergo a surgical termination of pregnancy at 10 weeks' gestation. Her sister died following a laparotomy for ectopic pregnancy, and she is concerned about her risk of death from the procedure.

Q9

Options:

A   Oral ofloxacin 400 mg bd plus oral metronidazole 400 mg bd for 7 days
B   Oral doxycycline 100 mg bd for 14 days
C   Oral ofloxacin 400 mg bd for 7 days
D   Oral ofloxacin 400 mg bd plus oral metronidazole 400 mg bd for 14 days
E   Intravenous cefuroxime 1.5 g tds and metronidazole 500 mg tds for 14 days
F   Remove IUCD plus oral ofloxacin 400 mg bd plus oral metronidazole 400 mg bd for 14 days
G   Oral erythromycin 250 mg qds for 7 days
H   Intravenous ofloxacin 400 mg bd plus intravenous metronidazole 500 mg tds for 14 days

I   Oral cefalexin 500 mg tds plus oral metronidazole 400 mg bd for 14 days
J   Oral erythromycin 500 mg qds for 7 days

Lead-in:

For each of the clinical presentations of genital tract infection below, please select *the most appropriate treatment* from the option list. Each option may be used once, more than once, or not at all.

Q41   A 17-year-old woman, who is using Depo-Provera® for contraception, presents with a five-day history of worsening lower abdominal pain and dyspareunia. On examination she looks generally well, but has lower abdominal and bilateral adnexal tenderness with positive cervical excitation.

Q42   A 22-year-old woman presents with lower abdominal pain and increased vaginal discharge for three weeks. She split up with her partner of two years five months ago. She has had several episodes of unprotected intercourse in this cycle but has not yet missed a period – this is due in five days. On examination she is apyrexial, she has lower abdominal and bilateral adnexal tenderness, and positive cervical excitation. Copious purulent cervical discharge is noted.

Q43   A 30-year-old woman, who is HIV positive, presents with acute lower abdominal pain. She has marked lower abdominal tenderness with guarding and a pelvic mass is suspected. She undergoes a laparotomy and drainage of a pelvic abscess.

Q44   A 19-year-old woman returns for medical advice; she presented one week ago with a two-week history of dyspareunia and pelvic pain, and was commenced on antibiotic treatment according to appropriate guidelines.

She is now complaining of worsening pain and a general feeling of malaise. On examination she appears flushed and is tachycardic; she has marked lower abdominal tenderness with guarding and rebound tenderness, and is exquisitely tender on vaginal examination.

(Q45) A 26-year-old woman, who has had an IUCD *in situ* for the past 18 months, presents with a seven-day history of lower abdominal pain and dyspareunia. Her LMP was one week ago. On examination she looks generally well, but has lower abdominal and bilateral adnexal tenderness with positive cervical excitation, and there is copious vaginal discharge.

Q10

Options:

A   Stop medication before trying to conceive
B   Adjust dose based on plasma drug level
C   Add new drug
D   Change to different drug
E   Reduce to monotherapy
F   Change route of administration
G   Change to slow-release preparation
H   Advise against pregnancy
I   Continue current treatment
J   Change class periconceptually and revert to original drug in second trimester

Lead-in:

For each of the women with chronic disease below, please select *the most appropriate pre-pregnancy advice* that might be offered by you in conjunction with the appropriate specialist. Each option may be used once, more than once, or not at all.

(Q46) You are asked to see a 37-year-old nulliparous woman for preconceptual counselling regarding her drug therapy. She has suffered from depressive illness for approximately eight years and is under the care of a psychiatrist. She has been hospitalised on two occasions, with the most recent episode being last year. She has been stable on clomipramine 100 mg nocte since that last episode. She got married three months ago and would like to start a family, however she is concerned that her medication might affect the baby and wants to stop it.

(Q47) A 29-year-old nulliparous woman is referred to you for pre-pregnancy advice. She has a large ASD which was diag-nosed one year ago after an acute hospital admission with breathlessness and syncope. You do not have her full cardiology record, but a recent ECG shows signs of right ventricular strain and a RBBB. She is currently on bosentan 125 mg daily and on warfarin, with an INR of approx-imately 2.

(Q48) A 40-year-old parous woman is referred to your pre-pregnancy clinic to discuss her medication prior to em-barking on a pregnancy. She was hospitalised under the Mental Health Act to prevent self-harm following a tragic accident 18 months ago when her husband of 15 years and their three children died in a house fire; she has since required treatment with paroxetine and is currently on 50 mg daily.

(Q49) A 21-year-old woman attends your preconceptual coun-selling clinic with her mother and her 19-year-old partner. She has suffered from grand-mal seizures since the age of 11. Her neurologist's letter suggests that her seizures were very difficult to control, and she had one acute admission with status epilepticus aged 15; however, she has been seizure free for five years on a combination of sodium valproate and lamotrigine.

Q50 A 40-year-old nulliparous woman with a BMI of 26 attends for preconceptual counselling. She has a strong family history of ischaemic heart disease, but no own history of any relevant symptoms. Her blood pressure has been marginally raised intermittently, but not high enough to warrant medication thus far. Her cholesterol level was borderline at her last check, and her GP started her on simvastatin.

Normal and complicated pregnancy

Q11

Options:

A   Threatened miscarriage
B   Biochemical pregnancy
C   Incomplete miscarriage
D   Septic miscarriage
E   Molar pregnancy
F   Choriocarcinoma
G   Missed miscarriage
H   Multiple pregnancy
I   Ectopic pregnancy
J   Normal intrauterine pregnancy

Lead-in:

For each of the early pregnancy scenarios described below, please select *the most likely diagnosis* from the option list. Each option may be used once, more than once, or not at all.

Q51   A 28-year-old woman undergoes IVF for tubal factor infertility. Two weeks after embryo transfer a blood test reveals a ßHCG of 98 iU/l and progesterone of 58 nmol/l. A repeat test 48 hours later shows a ßHCG of 210 iU/l and progesterone of 61 nmol/l; after a further 96 hours her serum ßHCG rises to 266 iU/l, whilst the progesterone level falls to15 nmol/l.

Q52 A 34-year-old woman undergoes medical TOP at eight weeks' gestation. She is readmitted seven days later with persistent lower abdominal pain and vaginal bleeding. On examination she has mild pyrexia of 37.2°C, lower abdominal tenderness and guarding. Pelvic ultrasound scan reports a mixed echogenic mass within the uterus measuring 1.4 × 2 cm. In the left adnexal region there is a mixed echogenic mass measuring 4 × 3.5 cm and a trace of fluid is seen in the POD. Both ovaries appear normal. Serum ßHCG on admission is 2139 iU/l; the level is 2270 iU/l 48 hours later.

Q53 A 29-year-old woman presents with vaginal bleeding following a 10-week history of amenorrhoea. A pelvic ultrasound demonstrates an intrauterine mixed echogenic mass of 4 × 5 cm, consistent with RPOC. She is treated with misoprostol and discharged home. One week later she is readmitted with heavy vaginal bleeding. Her temperature is 36.8°C, BP is 93/56 mmHg, and her pulse is 92 bpm. On examination the cervix admits a fingertip, and there is bilateral adnexal tenderness. Laboratory investigations reveal an Hb of 9.9 g/dl (11.5–16.5), WBC of 9 × 10^9/l (4–11), and a ßHCG of 3580 iU/l.

Q54 A 38-year-old woman, undergoing her fourth cycle of IVF, is admitted to hospital 28 days following embryo transfer with spotting per vaginam. She declines vaginal examination. Pelvic ultrasound scan demonstrates a 5 mm intra-uterine gestational sac, but no fetal pole could be identified. Her ßHCG is 19,800 iU/l.

Q55 A 25-year-old woman is admitted with lower abdominal pain and vaginal bleeding after seven weeks' amenorrhoea.

A pregnancy test is positive and a pelvic ultrasound scan reveals an empty uterus with a 1.5 × 2 cm cystic lesion in the left adnexum, and free fluid in the POD. She undergoes a diagnostic laparoscopy, which is negative. A ßHCG taken on the day of her laparoscopy is reported as 189 iU/l. This is repeated 42 hours later and is found to be 330 iU/l.

Q12

Options:

A   Administer 250 iU (50 mcg) anti-D immunoglobulin IM immediately, and perform Kleihauer-Bethke the following morning

B   Administer 500 iU (100 mcg) anti-D immunoglobulin IM immediately, and perform Kleihauer-Bethke the following morning

C   Administer 2500 iU (500 mcg) anti-D immunoglobulin IM immediately, and perform Kleihauer-Bethke the following morning

D   No need for anti-D immunoglobulin prophylaxis or Kleihauer-Bethke

E   Check Kleihauer-Bethke. No need for anti-D immunoglobulin

F   Check Kleihauer-Bethke within two hours. Administer 2500 iU anti-D immunoglobulin

G   Check Kleihauer-Bethke and administer 500 iU anti-D immunoglobulin

H   Administer 250 iU (50 mcg) anti-D immunoglobulin IM within 72 hours

I   Administer 500 iU (100 mcg) anti-D immunoglobulin IM within 72 hours

J   Administer 2500 iU (500 mcg) anti-D immunoglobulin IM within 72 hours

Lead-in:

For each of the rhesus-negative pregnant women below, please select *the most appropriate evidence-based management* from the option list. Each option may be used once, more than once, or not at all.

 An 18-year-old woman undergoes surgical TOP at eight weeks' gestation.

A 26-year-old woman is delivered by Caesarean section at 30 weeks' gestation because of severe IUGR. During antenatal screening she was found to have anti-Kell antibodies. At booking her anti-Kell titre was 1/64 and remained stable throughout pregnancy. Cord blood taken at delivery suggests that the baby is Rh positive.

A 34-year-old woman, whose family is complete and who was using an IUCD for contraception, undergoes laparoscopic left salpingectomy for an ectopic pregnancy, diagnosed following 6–7 weeks' amenorrhoea.

 A woman is involved in a road traffic accident at 22 weeks' gestation, and sustains a seat-belt injury to her abdomen. Fetal viability is confirmed on ultrasound.

A 23-year-old woman, who is a Jehovah's Witness, attends the antenatal clinic in her first pregnancy. Booking bloods reveal her rhesus status to be Cde/cde; her long-standing partner is also tested at her request and his rhesus status is cdE/CdE.

Q13

Options:

A Amniocentesis
B Chorionic villous sampling
C Fetal anomaly scan at 20–22 weeks' gestation
D 24-hour urinary VMA
E Glycosylated haemoglobin
F Hb electrophoresis
G Serum uric acid
H Oral glucose tolerance test
I Urinary protein/creatinine ratio
J Hepatitis serology
K Renal ultrasound
L Uterine artery Doppler
M Urine culture
N 24-hour ambulatory blood pressure measurement

Lead-in:

For each of the clinical presentations in pregnancy described below, please select *the single most useful test* from the option list. Each option may be used once, more than once, or not at all.

Q61 A 30-year-old primigravida attends for antenatal care at 18 weeks' gestation and is requesting a screening test for pre-eclampsia. She gives a family history of severe pre-eclampsia in her mother and sister. A dating ultrasound scan confirms her gestational age. Her BP in clinic is 115/60 mmHg.

Q62 A 36-year-old G2 P0 of Indo-Asian origin attends for routine antenatal care at 35 weeks' gestation. She complains of increasing abdominal discomfort over the past four weeks. Her parents are both diabetic. Her GP performed a random blood glucose test in the first trimester, which was normal. On examination her symphysio-fundal height is 40 cm. Ultrasound scan reveals both the fetal abdominal circumference and the amniotic fluid index to be above the 95th centile.

(Q63) A 33-year-old G3 P2 with two previous preterm deliveries presents for routine antenatal care at 32 weeks' gestation. Her blood pressure is 135/88 mmHg, and urinalysis reveals + protein, ++ leucocytes and ++ nitrites. You review her notes and find that she has had three positive MSU cultures in this pregnancy, all growing coliform bacilli.

(Q64) A 25-year-old woman attends for a serum Down syndrome screening blood test at 16 weeks' gestation. You review her notes and see that she has had asymptomatic bacteriuria at booking, which was treated with appropriate antibiotics. Subsequent urinalysis revealed + of protein and + of ketones on one occasion at 10 weeks' gestation, and a trace of protein and ++ of glucose at 12 weeks' gestation. Today her urinalysis is negative.

(Q65) A 30-year-old G2 P1, who had moderate pre-eclampsia in her last pregnancy, attends the antenatal clinic at 36 weeks' gestation. In this pregnancy her blood pressure has been normal. She is concerned as she has had some visual disturbances earlier in the day. On admission her blood pressure is 136/82 mmHg and there is + of protein on urinalysis.

Q14

Options:

A   Renal ultrasound scan
B   Stress test
C   Request fetal growth scan

D   Commence oral labetolol
E   Measure BP in 30-minute intervals
F   Hb electrophoresis
G   24-hour urine collection for protein quanitification
H   Administer oral atenolol
I   Administer oral hydralazine
J   Send an MSU sample for culture and sensitivity
K   Start intravenous magnesium sulphate
L   Administer intravenous labetolol

Lead-in:

For each of the following presentations of hypertension in pregnancy, please select *the most appropriate initial management* from the option list. Each option may be used once, more than once, or not at all.

(Q66)   A 21-year-old primigravida is admitted to the labour ward at 36 weeks' gestation with a headache, visual disturbances and epigastric pain. On admission her BP is140/80 mmHg and there are +++ of protein on urinalysis. Blood work reveals a platelet count of $120 \times 10^9/l$ (150–400), and an ALT 23 iU/l (10–50). The CTG is normal.

(Q67)   A 25-year-old primigravida attends the antenatal clinic at 29 weeks' gestation. Her BP is 140/90 mmHg (it was 110/70 mmHg at booking), and there are ++ of protein on urinalysis. The fetus is active and appropriately grown on clinical examination.

(Q68)   A 41-year-old parous woman presents for booking at 12 weeks' gestation. She has essential hypertension; she has discontinued her usual medication (lisinopril) when she found out she was pregnant. Her BP at presentation is 150/100 mmHg and urinalysis is negative.

(Q69) A 38-year-old primigravida presents to the labour ward at 37 weeks' gestation with a 48-hour history of right iliac fossa pain and irregular uterine tightenings. She has a long-standing history of renal disease and hypertension; during pregnancy her BP has been controlled on oral methyldopa 500 mg tds. On admission her blood pressure is 150/98 mmHg. There is + of protein on urinalysis.

(Q70) A 37-year-old G3 P2 attends the antenatal clinic at 32 weeks' gestation. She is pregnant as a result of IVF. Her booking BP was noted to be 140/88 mmHg, and a 24-hour ABPM was performed. This showed mean daytime reading of 121/72 mmHg, and a mean night-time reading of 102/53 mmHg. Because of recurrent glucosuria, a GTT was performed at 28 weeks' gestation. Her fasting glucose was 5.8 mmol/l, and the two hour value was 9.1 mmol/l. At presentation her BP is 140/90 mmHg, and urinalysis is clear.

Q15

Options:

A Central venous pressure catheter
B Transfusion with whole blood
C Transfusion with packed cells
D Cryoprecipitate administration
E Epidural analgesia
F Fetal blood sampling
G Emergency Caesarean section
H Urgent full blood count
I Platelet transfusion
J Intravenous antibiotics
K Heparinisation
L Oxygen by face mask
M Intravenous opiates
N Oxytocin augmentation

Lead-in:

For each of the following clinical presentations in pregnancy, please select *the single most important initial measure* in the management of the patient. Each option may be chosen once, more than once, or not at all.

(Q71) A 36-year-old primigravida, who has HbSC, is admitted at 38 weeks' gestation with a history of irregular contractions for the past 10 hours. The fetal membranes ruptured eight hours ago. On examination her cervix is 3 cm dilated, fully effaced and well applied to the presenting part. The fetus is presenting by the vertex, and the presenting part is at the level of the ischial spines. Her last FBC, taken 48 hours ago, revealed an Hb of 8.1 g/dl (11.5–16.5).

(Q72) A 20-year-old woman self-refers to the labour ward with lower abdominal pain. She is known to have HbSS and is currently 33 weeks pregnant. On examination she is mildly pyrexial, and appears pale and dehydrated. The symphysio-fundal height is 30 cm and the lie of the fetus is longitudinal. Urinalysis shows ++ of protein, + nitrites and + of blood. Her Hb is 7.5 g/dl (11.5–16.5).

(Q73) A 27-year-old with HbSC has an uneventful antenatal course, with a stable Hb of around 8.0 g/dl. She labours spontaneously at term and progresses to a normal vaginal delivery, with an estimated blood loss of 500 ml. Two hours postpartum she complains of breathlessness and palpitations. Her BP is recorded at 100/60 mmHg, and her pulse is 126 bpm. The uterus is well contracted but her urine output is poor. An FBC taken immediately after delivery reveals an Hb of 7.4 g/dl (11.5–16.5).

(Q74) A 21-year-old primigravida is admitted to the labour ward in early labour at 37 weeks' gestation. She is contracting regularly every 2–3 minutes and appears to be distressed. Her pregnancy has been uneventful; however it appears that she has not attended for antenatal care since her detailed scan at 20 weeks' gestation. Her FBC at booking revealed an Hb of 10.0 g/dl (11.5–16.5). On admission her BP is 116/67 mmHg, and her pulse is 100 bpm.

(Q75) A 26-year-old primigravida is admitted to the labour ward in labour at 39 weeks' gestation. She has been followed up in the high-risk antenatal clinic because of a history of ITP, and her last visit there was four hours before admission. Her platelets have remained at around $80 \times 10^9/l$ (150–400) during pregnancy, and the sample taken in clinic earlier today suggested no change. On admission her cervix is 8 cm dilated; the presenting part is at the level of the ischial spines, and the position is occipitotransverse. You are asked to see her because of persistent late decelerations and reduced baseline variability on the CTG.

Q16

Options:

A   Uterine artery Doppler velocimetry
B   Induction of labour
C   Twice-weekly cardiotocography
D   Vena cava Doppler velocimetry
E   Caesarean section
F   Weekly umbilical artery Doppler velocimetry
G   Daily cardiotocography
H   Amniocentesis
I   Daily middle cerebral artery Doppler velocimetry
J   Ductus venosus Doppler velocimetry

Lead-in:

For each of the following cases of suspected fetal growth restriction, please select *the most appropriate management* from the option list. Each option may be used once, more than once, or not at all.

(Q76) A 29-year-old primigravida with a BMI of 30 presents to the labour ward with reduced fetal movements at 35 weeks' gestation. On examination her BP is 144/90 mmHg and urinalysis reveals + of proteinuria. Ultrasound assessment suggests an HC on the 5th centile, AC below the 3rd centile, with an amniotic fluid index on the 5th centile. Umbilical artery Doppler velocimetry demonstrates absent end-diastolic flow, and the middle cerebral artery Doppler flow is appropriate for the gestation. Admission CTG is normal.

(Q77) A 17-year-old primigravida with a BMI of 19 is referred by her community midwife to the antenatal clinic at 25 weeks' gestation with a symphysio-fundal height of 22 cm. Her BP is 133/78 mmHg, and urinalysis is negative. Ultrasound reveals an HC and AC below the 3rd centile. AFI is on the 5th centile. Umbilical artery Doppler reveals reversed end-diastolic flow and there is evidence of compensatory flow in the middle cerebral artery.

(Q78) A 45-year-old parous woman with a BMI of 33 presents to the antenatal clinic at 38 weeks' gestation because of lack of increase in her symphysio-fundal height over four weeks, according to her midwife's assessment. Her BP is 128/77 mmHg, and urinalysis is negative. Ultrasound assessment suggests an HC on the 30th and an AC on the 5th centile, AFI is below the 3rd centile. Umbilical artery Doppler velocimetry is appropriate for gestation.

(Q79) A 33-year-old primigravida is referred to the antenatal clinic at 27 weeks' gestation because of a symphysio-fundal height of 23 cm. Her BP is 132/88 mmHg, and there is a trace of protein on urinalysis. Ultrasound suggests an

HC and an AC below the 3rd centile and an AFI on the 97th centile. Umbilical artery Doppler reveals a continuous end-diastolic flow.

(Q80) A 22-year-old Para 1 is admitted with suspected fetal growth restriction at 27 weeks' gestation. On admission her BP is 110/65 mmHg, urinalysis is negative. Ultrasound reveals an HC on the 7th centile, an AC below the 3rd centile, and an AFI on the 5th centile. There is reversed end-diastolic flow in the umbilical artery, and the middle cerebral artery flow is appropriate for gestation.

Intrapartum care

Q17

Options:

A   Moriceau-Smellie-Veit manoeuvre
B   Rubin's manoeuvre
C   Heimlich manoeuvre
D   Brand-Andrews manoeuvre
E   McRoberts manoeuvre
F   Lövset's manoeuvre
G   Credé manoeuvre
H   Prague manoeuvre
I   Bracht manoeuvre
J   Pajot manoeuvre
K   Breech extraction
L   Zavanelli manoeuvre

Lead-in:

For each of the intrapartum scenarios below, please select *the most appropriate obstetric manoeuvre* from the option list. Each option may be used once, more than once, or not at all.

 A 32-year-old G3 P1, who has previously had a normal vaginal delivery of a male infant weighing 4.5 kg, is admitted in spontaneous labour. The present pregnancy has been uncomplicated, and on ultrasound assessment the fetal growth has been along the 50th centile. She has had an epidural block sited and finds it difficult to generate effective expulsive effort. You wish to perform a Neville-Barnes forceps delivery for delay in second stage of labour. On examination there are 0/5 palpable per abdomen; the patient's cervix is fully dilated and her membranes are absent. The fetus is presenting by the vertex in DOA position. The station of the presenting part is at the ischial spines, with minimal caput and reducible moulding.

(Q82) You are conducting a term vaginal breech delivery on a 41-year-old primigravida. On admission to the labour ward her cervix was found to be fully dilated and the breech was on the perineum. The midwife called you urgently, and on arrival you find the patient in lithotomy position; the body of the fetus has now delivered and the baby is hanging by the head in a sacroposterior position.

(Q83) You have been summoned by the alarm bell to a delivery room. A singleton term delivery is in progress. The fetal head has delivered two contractions ago, but there is difficulty with the shoulders. The midwife has hyperflexed the mother's hips before the last contraction, and a second midwife has applied suprapubic pressure, but this has not been successful.

(Q84) You are conducting a term twin delivery on a 22-year-old primigravida. The first twin delivered spontaneously from a vertex presentation. The second twin, who appears to be bigger than the first, is presenting by the breech. The membranes rupture spontaneously with the breech on the perineum, and the body of the fetus delivers over a further two contractions to the level of the inferior scapular angle.

(Q85) You are conducting a term vaginal breech delivery on a 33-year-old multipara, who declined external cephalic version or Caesarean section. She laboured spontaneously and made good progress in labour. You were called when the breech was visible at the introitus; on your arrival you find that the body of the fetus has delivered and the baby is now hanging by the head in the sacroanterior position.

Q18

Options:

A   Fetal blood sampling
B   Emergency Caesarean section grade 1
C   Emergency Caesarean section grade 3
D   Continuous external fetal monitoring
E   Continuous internal fetal monitoring
F   Augment labour
G   Discontinue oxytocin infusion
H   Forceps delivery using Wrigley's forceps
I   Forceps delivery using Kjelland's forceps
J   Forceps delivery using Neville-Barnes forceps
K   Ventouse delivery using silastic cup
L   Ventouse delivery using metal OP cup
M   External cephalic version

Lead-in:

For each of the following intrapartum case scenarios, please select *the single best management option* from the option list. Each option may be used once, more than once, or not at all.

 A 30-year-old primigravida with a booking BMI of 29 is admitted to the labour ward at 28 weeks' gestation with intermittent abdominal pain and moderate vaginal bleeding. On clinical examination the uterus is about 30 weeks in size, and there is mild uterine tenderness. The cervix is fully dilated and membranes are absent; the fetus is presenting by the breech and bloodstained liquor is noted. The fetal heart rate is auscultated at 154 bpm, and no decelerations were noted.

Q87 A 39-year-old parous woman with IDDM is admitted to the labour ward complaining of intermittent abdominal pain and a 'show' at 34^{+5} weeks' gestation. Her BMI at booking was 32. She had regular antenatal care and the fetus appears appropriately grown. During the antenatal course her diabetic control was difficult, and on admission her blood sugar is 10.5 mmol/l. On auscultation of the fetal heart a deceleration to 80 bpm is audible, but this recovers by the end of the contraction. The cervix is fully dilated, and the presentation is cephalic, in LOA position. The presenting part is at the level of the ischial spines and 0/5 are palpable per abdomen.

Q88 A 23-year-old Para 2 undergoes IOL at 39 weeks' gestation because of pre-eclampsia. Her BP has been mildly to moderately raised, and she has 3 g of protein in a 24-hour urine collection. Her BMI is 35. The fetal membranes are ruptured artificially at 2 cm dilatation and oxytocin infusion is commenced. Contractions are maintained at a frequency of 1:3. On examination six hours later the cervix was noted to be 7 cm dilated. After a further six hours the patient reaches full cervical dilatation, the presenting part is at the ischial spines in LOA position, with 0/5 of the head palpable abdominally. There is no significant caput or moulding. You are called to see her as variable decelerations are noted on the CTG over a period of 30 minutes following the vaginal examination. The fetal heart rate is 165 bpm, and the baseline variability is 4 bpm.

Q89 A 39-year-old Para 5 is admitted in spontaneous labour. She requests a regional block for analgesia, and this is sited without complications. Full cervical dilatation is documented six hours after admission and active second stage is commenced 45 minutes later. One hour later medical review is requested; 0/5 is palpable abdominally, the cervix is again noted to be fully dilated, the presenting part is at the level of the ischial spines in ROP position, with + of caput and no moulding. CTG shows decelerations down to 50 bpm, which occur synchronously with contractions. There is normal baseline variability.

(Q90) A 28-year-old HIV-positive woman with a viral load of 50 copies/ml is admitted at 38 weeks' gestation with irregular contractions. On admission her cervix is found to be 2 cm dilated and the membranes are absent. The presenting part is cephalic, with 3/5 palpable per abdomen. Auscultation of the fetal heart rate showed a baseline of 150 bpm, with no audible decelerations following contractions.

Q19

Options:

A   Mid-cavity forceps
B   Low forceps
C   Outlet forceps
D   Ventouse extraction
E   Encourage maternal effort
F   Caesarean section
G   Atosiban administration
H   Oxytocin augmentation
I   Mobilisation
J   Rehydration

Lead-in:

For each of the following intrapartum scenarios, please select *the most appropriate management* from the option list. Each option may be used once, more than once, or not at all.

Q91 A 31-year-old primigravida with long-standing IDDM is admitted in spontaneous labour at 34 weeks' gestation. On examination a long lie and cephalic presentation are noted, and clinically the baby appears to be appropriately grown. Her cervix is 4 cm dilated; continuous electronic fetal monitoring is commenced. Sliding-scale insulin infusion is commenced and epidural analgesia is administered at her request. Four hours later variable decelerations are noted on the CTG. On examination the cervix is fully dilated and the membranes are noted to be absent; the fetus is presenting by the vertex, in direct occipitoanterior position, with the presenting part at the level of the ischial spines +2. There is a loop of cord palpable adjacent to the fetal head on the right.

Q92 A 34-year-old primigravida is admitted in spontaneous labour at 39 weeks' gestation. Clinical examination suggests an average size fetus in a cephalic presentation; the cervix is 2 cm dilated and the membranes are absent. Epidural block is sited and an oxytocin infusion is commenced because contractions become infrequent. Continuous electronic fetal monitoring is in progress. After a further eight hours she is found to be fully dilated, and an ARM is performed. One hour later, vaginal examination is repeated; the presenting part is at the level of the ischial spines +2, and the position is left occipitotransverse. The presenting part is not palpable per abdomen.

Q93 A 17-year-old primigravida is admitted to the labour ward in advanced labour following a concealed pregnancy of unknown gestation. She is extremely distressed and an epidural has to be sited prior to vaginal examination. Clinical examination reveals a uterine size compatible with approximately 34 weeks' gestation. On vaginal examination her cervix is 9 cm dilated; the fetus is presenting by the vertex in direct occipitoposterior position, and the presenting part is the level of the spines. Continuous fetal monitoring is satisfactory. Two hours later full cervical dilatation is confirmed, the presenting part has rotated to DOA position and descended below the ischial spines (station 0+2). None of the presenting part is palpable per abdomen. Progress in the second stage is slow, and two hours later she remains undelivered.

Q94   A 30-year-old G3 P2, who has booked a planned home birth, is transferred to the labour ward by her midwife because of delay in the second stage of labour. On admission the attending midwife advises that the patient has been fully dilated for three hours, despite rapid progress in the first stage. Uterine contractions are now occurring at a frequency of 2/10. On examination the cervix is fully dilated and membranes are absent. The fetus is presenting by the vertex in DOP position, the presenting part is at the level of the ischial spines −1.

Q95   A 33-year-old primigravida is admitted in spontaneous labour at 37 weeks' gestation. Her pregnancy has been uncomplicated; she has a long-standing history of ITP, however her platelet count has been normal in pregnancy. On examination her cervix is noted to be 5 cm dilated, and full cervical dilatation is achieved four hours later. She is using entonox for analgesia. After two hours in the second stage she remains undelivered. On examination there is 0/5 palpable per abdomen, the presenting part is noted to be at the level of the spines +1 and in DOA position.

Q20

Options:

A   Await spontaneous labour
B   Elective Caesarean section
C   Elective instrumental delivery
D   Induction of labour at 37 weeks' gestation
E   Induction of labour at 40 weeks' gestation
F   Elective episiotomy
G   Short trial of labour with early recourse to emergency Caesarean section
H   Encourage to deliver in all-fours position
I   Avoid epidural anaesthesia
J   Decide on mode of delivery based on fetal ultrasound at 40 weeks' gestation

Lead-in:

For each of the following pregnancy histories, please select *the most appropriate evidence-based advice* from the option list. Each option may be used once, more than once, or not at all.

Q96 A 33-year-old G3 P1 with a booking BMI of 32 attends the high-risk antenatal clinic at 20 weeks' gestation to discuss her delivery. In her last pregnancy she went into spontaneous labour at 38 weeks' gestation and had a vaginal delivery, but unfortunately this was complicated by shoulder dystocia. She delivered a live male infant weighing 3895 g, who developed neonatal encephalopathy. The child is left with neuro-developmental problems and persistent Erb's palsy.

Q97 A 26-year-old primigravida with a booking BMI of 29, who has diet-controlled gestational diabetes mellitus, attends the obstetric-diabetic clinic at 36 weeks' gestation for a routine visit. Her blood sugar home monitoring shows capillary glucose results ranging from 3.6–6.9 mmol/l over the past two weeks. Her urinalysis is negative for glucose. An ultrasound performed two days ago shows fetal head circumference on the 90th and abdominal circumference on the 85th centile, with an amniotic fluid index on the 75th centile.

Q98 A 40-year-old G2 P0 with a booking BMI of 26 is referred to the high-risk antenatal clinic at 39 weeks' gestation because the midwife was concerned about her fundal height. An ultrasound assessment suggests an estimated fetal weight of 4450 g, with an amniotic fluid index on the 90th centile.

Q99 A 25-year-old primigravida with a 10-year history of IDDM attends the obstetric-diabetic clinic at 36 weeks' gestation following an ultrasound assessment of fetal growth. This suggests fetal head circumference on the 90th centile, and the abdominal circumference is above the 95th centile. Amniotic fluid index is above the 95th centile.

Q100 A 37-year-old G3 P2 attends a high-risk antenatal clinic at 20 weeks' gestation to discuss her delivery. In her first pregnancy she was induced at 38 weeks' gestation for raised BP and underwent a Kjelland's forceps delivery in theatre; this was complicated by shoulder dystocia and extensive perineal trauma. She delivered a live female infant weighing 3670 g; the baby spent 12 hours on the neonatal unit and was then discharged to the postnatal ward. There was mild left-sided Erb's palsy which resolved by the age of three weeks. In her second pregnancy she went into spontaneous labour at term and had a normal, uncomplicated vaginal delivery of a male weighing 4600 g.

General gynaecology

Q21

Options:

A Endometrial polyp
B Atrophic endometrium
C Luteal phase defect
D Poorly differentiated endometrial carcinoma
E Arias-Stella reaction
F Early secretory endometrium
G Well-differentiated endometrial carcinoma
H Late proliferative endometrium
I Late secretory endometrium
J Inadequate sample
K Early proliferative endometrium
L Endometrial hyperplasia
M Dyssynchronous secretory endometrium

Lead-in:

For each of the following cases, please select *the most appropriate histological diagnosis* from the option list. Each option may be used once, more than once, or not at all.

Q101 A 70-year-old woman presents following an episode of postmenopausal bleeding. Hysteroscopy reveals a normal uterine cavity. The endometrium is macroscopically unremarkable. The histology report reads as follows: *There is little material in the sample received. This shows sparse narrow glands lined by a low epithelium with small nuclei. The stoma is dense and fibrous with spindle cells.*

Q102 A 40-year-old woman attends the gynaecology clinic because of irregular, prolonged periods. She has been taking medication to regulate her cycles as advised by her GP; however she can't recall the name of the drug. She undergoes endometrial biopsy 20 days into therapy. The histology report reads as follows: *The endometrium exhibits few thin endometrial glands. The glands are poorly developed, some containing subnuclear vacuoles, others containing abortive secretions. The surrounding stroma is abundant, with localised areas where stromal cells are enlarged and circular, containing clear cytoplasm surrounding central vesicular nuclei.*

Q103 A 30-year-old woman presents with irregular vaginal bleeding and left iliac fossa pain. Her urinary pregnancy test is weakly positive. Her serum ßHCG rose from 155 iU/l to 231 iU/l over 48 hours. She passes a piece of 'tissue' which is sent for histological diagnosis. The histology report reads as follows: *The glands are closely packed and appear hypersecretory. The glandular epithelial cells appear hyperchromatic with large irregular nuclei. The superficial layer of the endometrial stroma exhibits large polygonal cells with a wide zone of cytoplasm surrounding the nucleus.*

Q104 A 25-year-old woman is being investigated for anovulatory infertility. She has been on clomiphene citrate for three cycles, but her cycles are short (bleeding on days 25–27). She undergoes endometrial biopsy. The histology report reads as follows: *The specimen consists mainly of blood* *with few fragments of endometrium. The endometrial glands are poorly grown, presenting straight or coiled narrow-calibre tubular profiles lined by epithelium that in some areas appears inactive but elsewhere features supra- and subnuclear secretory vacuoles. The stroma is mildly oedematous and non-decidualised, showing areas of breakdown.*

 A 45-year-old woman with PCOS undergoes endometrial sampling because of recent onset of irregular vaginal bleeding. In the past she had periods of amenorrhoea of up to six months, but had declined hormonal treatment because of side-effects. The histology report reads as follows: *This is a good sample of endometrium. The glands are dilated and cystic, of irregular size and shape. The glandular epithelium is pseudostratified columnar and shows numerous mitoses. Nuclei are oval with smooth contours, evenly dispersed chromatin, and small, inconspicuous nucleoli. In areas, there is a reduced stroma-to-glandular ratio.*

Q22

Options:

A   Microwave endometrial ablation
B   Thermal balloon endometrial ablation
C   Tranexamic acid
D   Expectant management
E   Myomectomy
F   Uterine artery embolisation
G   Total abdominal hysterectomy and bilateral salpingo-oophorectomy
H   GnRH analogues
I   Hysteroscopic myomectomy
J   Mirena® intrauterine system
K   TAH
L   Radio-ablation of ovaries

Lead-in:

For each of the clinical presentations of uterine fibroids below, please select *the most appropriate management option* from the option list. Each option can be used once, more than once, or not at all.

Q106   A 38-year-old parous African woman presents with heavy periods and dysmenorrhoea. She has not used contraception for the last four years whilst trying for a pregnancy. Her periods are very heavy with flooding and large clots. Her Hb is 7.5 g/dl (11.5–16.5). Her GP identified a fibroid uterus and arranged a pelvic ultrasound scan. This reported the uterus to be $10.5 \times 5 \times 4.5$ cm, containing multiple echogenic areas of 2 cm maximum diameter.

Q107   A 36-year-old nulliparous woman presents with heavy periods. Her GP has tried several types of drugs, but these have not been effective. Clinical examination reveals a 10 weeks' size fibroid uterus. Pelvic ultrasound scan reports an enlarged uterus of $11 \times 6 \times 5$ cm, with the endometrial cavity distorted by a 3×2.5 cm mass, possibly a fibroid. Subsequent hysteroscopy demonstrates a grade 1 submucous fibroid.

Q108   A 34-year-old parous woman who has had three Caesarean sections and a tubal ligation presents with heavy periods; she has been forced to take time off work and curtail her usual activities, including taking her young children swimming. Her GP has tried several types of drugs, but she has not been able to tolerate these because of gastro-intestinal side-effects. Clinical examination is uninformative because of her BMI. Pelvic ultrasound scan suggests a possible small fibroid, but overall uterine dimensions, which could only be ascertained with difficulty, are $8.5 \times 5 \times 4$ cm. Subsequent hysteroscopy demonstrates a normal uterine cavity of 11 cm sound length and a small posterior-wall intra-mural fibroid.

(Q109) A 28-year-old nulliparous African woman presents with heavy periods associated with flooding, clots and infertility. On examination she has a pelvi-abdominal mass of about 20 weeks' size, consistent with a fibroid uterus. Three years previously she had a midline laparotomy in her native Zimbabwe, which resulted in a bowel injury due to extensive adhesions of uncertain cause. You request an ultrasound scan which suggests a fibroid uterus.

(Q110) A 24-year-old parous African woman attends the gynaecology clinic at six weeks postpartum. She had no difficulty getting pregnant, but was noted at her antenatal booking scan to have multiple uterine fibroids. She was delivered by elective Caesarean section at 38 weeks' gestation because of a cervical fibroid obstructing the birth canal. She is still breast-feeding and has not resumed her periods. On examination the uterus is enlarged to 16 weeks' size and there is a posterior cervical fibroid of about 6 cm diameter.

Q23

Options:

A   Oral metoclopramide 10 mg tds
B   Goserelin acetate 3.6 mg injection every 28 days
C   Cetrorelix 250 mcg SC injection
D   Gestrinone 2.5 mg twice per week
E   Oral paracetamol 1g qds
F   Medroxyprogesterone acetate 10mg tds
G   Mefenamic acid 500 mg tds
H   Reassurance and support
I   Oral mebeverine 200 mg bd
J   Levonorgestrel IUS
K   Ethinylestradiol + drospirenone
L   Diagnostic laparoscopy

M Laparotomy
N TAH and BSO

Lead-in:

For each of the following case scenarios with pelvic pain, please select *the most suitable management* from the option list. Each option may be used once, more than once, or not at all.

(Q111)   A 30-year-old nulliparous woman with a BMI of 28, who is currently using Depo-Provera® for contraception, is referred by her GP because of persistent pelvic pain. She has had symptoms of pain for several years, but has experienced an increase in severity over the past 12 months. The pain is present for most of the cycle, with premenstrual exacerbation and some improvement following menses. Additionally, there is some dyspareunia which may persist following intercourse. Analgesics have failed to control the symptoms. Clinical examination revealed bilateral adnexal tenderness but no masses.

(Q112)   A 38-year-old Para 4 with a BMI of 22, who underwent laparoscopic sterilisation two years ago, presents with recurrent lower abdominal pain over the past seven months. The pain is not related to her cycle and it can occur at any time – on average she has experienced it once a week. It has not impacted on her daily activities, but the patient is concerned about what might be causing it. There is no dysmenorrhoea, dyspareunia or bowel/urinary symptoms. On examination her uterus is anteverted and mobile; the adnexa appear normal and there is no pelvic tenderness.

(Q113)   A 27-year-old nulliparous woman with a BMI of 29 presents with a three-year history of cyclical pelvic pain. She is not sexually active. She complains of lethargy, bloating and painful defaecation, particularly during her periods. Her bowel habits have never been regular and she has a tendency to constipation. There are no urinary symptoms. On examination she appears healthy. Abdominal examination reveals tenderness in the left iliac fossa. The uterus is of normal size, anteverted, and there is some tenderness in the POD.

(Q114) A 35-year-old G3 P2 with a BMI of 30 suffered a bowel injury at the time of a TOP, which required a laparotomy and right hemicolectomy. Two years later she presents with an ongoing history of pelvic and abdominal pain, and dyspareunia; her symptoms appear to be worsening. There is constant central and lower abdominal pain associated with anorexia and abdominal distension. There is no clear link to the menstrual cycle. During acute exacerbations the pain becomes severe, requiring bed rest, and can be associated with nausea and vomiting.

(Q115) A 17-year-old nulliparous woman with a BMI of 19 presents with pelvic pain. Her pain is cyclical, starting a few days prior to her period, and is completely relieved within 36–48 hours of onset of bleeding. She had Implanon® inserted for contraception following a TOP one year ago. You note that at the time of TOP she tested positive for chlamydia, but there is uncertainty as to whether she received treatment. Over-the-counter medication has not helped. Clinical examination is normal apart from mild tenderness of the left adnexum.

Q24

Options:

A   Laparoscopic ovarian cystectomy
B   Diagnostic laparoscopy
C   Ultrasound guided biopsy
D   Transvaginal ultrasound scan
E   Danazol
F   COCP
G   IVF
H   LNG-IUS
I   Letrozole
J   Ablation of endometriotic lesion
K   Unilateral oophorectomy
L   TAH and BSO
M   Uterine nerve ablation
N   IUI

Lead-in:

For each of the following cases, please select *the most appropriate management* from the option list. Each option may be used once, more than once, or not at all.

(Q116)   A 28-year-old nulliparous woman with a BMI of 23 presents with a history of dysmenorrhoea and dyspareunia. The pain starts a few days prior to the onset of bleeding. She has experienced some pain since menarche at the age of 13, but the symptoms have become worse since she stopped the oral contraceptive pill one year ago whilst trying to conceive. Clinical examination reveals bilateral adnexal tenderness; there are no masses or nodules in the POD but there is tenderness in the posterior fornix. Her past history includes a diagnostic laparoscopy five years ago for suspected appendicitis.

Q117 A 31-year-old nulliparous woman with a BMI of 22 presents with a three-year history of primary infertility. She is otherwise asymptomatic. Clinical examination reveals a fixed left adnexal mass of approximately 5 cm diameter. The uterus is fixed and retroverted, but of normal size. An ultrasound scan confirms a complex left adnexal mass. Subsequent investigations reveal grade IV endometriosis.

Q118 A 36-year-old nulliparous woman with a BMI of 28 presents with a long history of pelvic pain and dyspareunia. Despite multiple analgesic agents, her symptoms remain disabling and result in frequent absence from work. Dyspareunia is severe and the patient avoids intercourse most of the month. She is determined to remain childless and has used reversible long-acting contraception for the past eight years. Clinical examination reveals a right adnexal mass of approximately 4 cm diameter. The uterus is of normal size and fixed. Further investigations reveal stage III endometriosis.

Q119 A 29-year-old nulliparous woman with a BMI of 32 presents with a four-year history of severe dysmenorrhoea. The pain starts a few days prior to the onset of bleeding and is present during the period. Multiple attempts at medical therapy, including oral and injectable hormonal preparations, have been unsuccessful. There is no dyspareunia. Clinical examination reveals bilateral adnexal tenderness but no pelvic masses. Her past history includes a diagnostic laparoscopy for suspected ectopic pregnancy, when endometriosis was noted on the right ovary which was densely adherent to the posterior leaf of the broad ligament.

Q120 A 30-year-old Para 1 with a BMI of 32 and a long-standing history of endometriosis attends the gynaecology clinic with recurrence of cyclical pelvic pain and dyspareunia; endometriosis was successfully treated in the past with medication. She is complaining of pain a few days prior to onset of menstruation, but the most severe symptoms occur during the first three days of the menses, improving when the flow lightens on day 4. Analgesia proved ineffective. Her only child was born by Caesarean section two years ago, and she is planning another pregnancy in a year or two. She takes propranolol for migraine and prednisolone for ulcerative colitis, although this has been quiescent recently.

Q25

Options:

A Injury to the jejunum and ileum
B Bladder perforation
C Ureteric ligation
D Perforation of the rectum
E Injury to the internal iliac vessels
F Injury to the inferior epigastric artery
G Uterine perforation
H Injury to the vaginal wall
I Vaginal stenosis
J Urinary retention
K Osteomalacia

Lead-in:

For each of the following cases, please select *the most relevant complication* from the option list. Each option may be used once, more than once, or not at all.

 A 64-year-old woman undergoes diagnostic hysteroscopy for postmenopausal bleeding. The uterine cavity has an atrophic appearance and contains a small polyp. Polypectomy is attempted, and the ovum forceps was introduced to a depth of about 12 cm.

 Q122 An 18-year-old woman is undergoing suction termination of pregnancy at 10 weeks' gestation. A size 6 Hegar dilator is introduced through the cervix to a depth of 14 cm; this is followed by brisk bleeding.

 Q123 A 60-year-old woman undergoes a procedure to treat urinary stress incontinence. The operation is performed under spinal anaesthesia.

 Q124 A 43-year-old woman undergoes microwave ablation of the endometrium for heavy periods. The procedure appears uneventful, but she is readmitted two days after surgery with abdominal distension and vomiting. She is apyrexial and the leukocyte count is normal.

Q125 A 24-year-old woman with dyspareunia undergoes laparoscopic resection of endometriosis in the rectovaginal septum. The procedure is performed via four access ports. During surgery the operative field becomes contaminated with faecal matter.

Q26

Options:

A Lichen sclerosus
B Seborrhoeic dermatitis
C Atopic vulvitis
D Lichen simplex
E Psoriasis
F Herpes simplex
G Behçet's disease
H Hidradenitis suppurativa

I   Paget's disease
J   Tinea cruris

Lead-in:

For each of the following patients with vulval symptoms, please select *the most likely* diagnosis from the list. Each option may be used once, more than once, or not at all.

Q126   A five-year-old girl presents with burning on micturition and vulval scratching. On examination the vulva is noted to have a well-demarcated white area around the introitus. The overlying skin appears thin with extensive fissuring. The peri-anal area is not involved.

Q127   A 70-year-old postmenopausal woman presents with vulval itching. On examination, she has a narrow introitus. The skin over the labia, perineal area and the genitocrural folds is thin, dry, with white discoloration and superficial excoriations. A skin biopsy reveals atrophic epidermis with hyperkeratosis, and superficial dermal hyalinisation with lymphocytic infiltrates.

Q128   A 65-year-old woman presents with long-standing vulval pruritus. On examination the labia major and surrounding perineal skin is noted to be erythematous. The skin is thickened, but with areas of excoriation secondary to itching. Histological examination of a skin biopsy showed parakeratosis and papillomatosis. There is no apparent neutrophil infiltrate in the epidermis.

Q129   A 23-year-old woman presents with vulval itching. On examination there is a well-demarcated symmetrical lesion involving the labia major and minor and extending to the genitocrural folds. The lesions appear beefy-red with scaling. A biopsy shows papillomatosis, parakeratosis and neutrophil exocytosis.

 A 34-year-old woman presents with a burning sensation in the vulval region. On examination the vulva is erythematous with marked oedema and numerous small superficial ulcerations. The inguinal lymph nodes are enlarged and tender.

Endocrinology and infertility

Q27

Options:

A   Antithyroid antibodies
B   Urinary metanephrine
C   Fasting plasma glucose
D   Serum prolactin
E   Midday plasma cortisol
F   Urinary 17-hydroxycorticosteroids
G   24-hour urinary-free cortisol
H   CRH stimulation test
I   17-hydroxyprogesterone (17-OHP)
J   ACTH stimulation test
K   Reverse T3
L   GnRH stimulation test

Lead-in:

For each of the following clinical presentations, please select *the single most useful test* from the option list. Each option may be used once, more than once, or not at all.

(Q131)   A 23-year-old nulliparous woman is referred to the gynaecology clinic because of infrequent menstruation and

excessive hair growth. She has periods of amenorrhoea lasting up to four months; when bleeding does occur it usually lasts 2–5 days. She has always been overweight, however she has experienced increased weight gain recently; her BMI is currently 38, and she has developed multiple striae on her breasts and abdomen. Additionally, she is complaining of increased facial hair growth as well as excess hair on her arms, breasts and back. Pelvic examination is uninformative because of her habitus. Transvaginal ultrasound demonstrates a normal uterus; the right ovary contained three small cysts, the largest being 5 mm in diameter.

Q132 A 42-year-old parous woman presents with a four-year history of irregular heavy periods. Prior to that she had used the COCP for approximately 12 years. Her current cycle pattern is 5–7/22–36. There is no intermenstrual or postcoital bleeding. Physical examination is grossly normal, and her BP is 130/82 mmHg. Her GP had sent a blood test for a hormone profile, which revealed the following results: FSH 11 mU/l (1–20), LH 13.2 mU/l (1–20), T4 12 pmol/l (9–24), T3 5 pmol/l (3–9 pmol/l) and TSH 7.5 mU/l (0.4–4.8 mU/l). Cholesterol was 5.7 mmol/l (<5.5 mmol/l), triglycerides 1.7 mmol/l (<2.0 mmol/l).

Q133 A 19-year-old nulliparous woman presents to the gynaecology clinic because of infrequent periods. She has only had six periods since menarche at age 15. The bleeding may last 1–2 days, often only as spotting. On examination she is obese with a BMI of 37, with striae on her abdomen and breasts. Breast development is Tanner stage 5. Excessive facial hair is also present. Her blood pressure is 135/85 mmHg. She declines pelvic examination. Transvaginal ultrasound demonstrates a normal uterus; the right ovary contains one cystic lesion measuring 3 mm in diameter.

Q134 A 35-year-old woman is undergoing investigations for oligomenorrhoea and obesity. She is found to have raised levels of urinary and plasma cortisol.

A 37-year-old parous woman with a BMI of 23 presents with secondary amenorrhoea of two years' duration. Her periods have been regular till the normal birth of her last child. She breast-fed her baby for four months, but had only one period when she stopped breast-feeding and has remained amenorrhoeic since. There is no galactorrhoea. She takes venlafaxine regularly, and occasional paracetamol for headaches. Clinical examination is normal.

Q28

Options:

A   Hyperaldosteronism
B   Diabetes insipidus
C   Anorexia nervosa
D   Hyperthyroidism
E   Bulimia
F   Kallman's syndrome
G   Congenital adrenal hyperplasia
H   Pheochromocytoma
I   Conn syndrome
J   Polycystic ovary syndrome
K   Craniopharyngioma
L   Prolactinoma
M   Cushing syndrome
N   Sheehan's syndrome
O   Diabetes mellitus

Lead-in:

For each of the clinical presentations described below, please select *the single most likely diagnosis* from the option list. Each option may be used once, more than once, or not at all.

(Q136) A 33-year-old woman with a BMI of 22 presents with primary infertility of four years' duration. She also complains of recurrent attacks of throbbing headaches, usually accompanied by sweating, palpitations and tremors. She suffers from these episodes almost 2–3 times per month. During the last episode, the headache was severe and she called out her GP, who documented an unremarkable physical examination except for a raised BP. The GP ascribes this to her anxiety about her infertility. In between episodes, she is asymptomatic and her BP is normal.

(Q137) A 28-year-old woman with a BMI of 29 presents with primary infertility of 24 months' duration. She experiences occasional headaches but is otherwise well apart from occasionally missing periods. She is normotensive. Her hormonal profile is as follows: FSH 3.5 iU/l (1–20), LH 6.4 iU/l (1–20), prolactin 1790 mU/l (50–500), free T4 14 pmol/L (9–25), TSH 3.4 mU/l (0.4–3). An ultrasound scan of her pelvis shows multiple follicles in both ovaries, the largest measuring 14 mm.

(Q138) A 29-year-old nulliparous woman presents to the gynaecology clinic because her periods have been infrequent for the past two years, occurring every 4–6 months. The bleeding may last up to two days, often only as spotting. On examination she is obese with a BMI of 37, with striae on her abdomen and breasts. Her blood pressure is 140/88 mmHg. She declines pelvic examination, but agrees to a transvaginal ultrasound scan which demonstrates a normal uterus; the right ovary contains one cyst measuring 3 mm in diameter.

(Q139)   A 33-year-old nulliparous woman with a BMI of 38 presents with a two-year history of oligomenorrhoea. She stopped the COCP two years ago in order to conceive, but her periods have been very infrequent since, only occurring every 4–6 months. There is no galactorrhoea or hirsutism. Clinical examination is normal. A hormone profile reveals the following: FSH 2.9 iU/ml (1–20), LH 13.1 iU/ml (1–20), TSH 4.5 mU/l (0.3–4), prolactin 655 mU/l (50–500). Free androgen index is 4.6% (3–7). Her fasting glucose is 5.8 mmol/l, two-hour postprandial glucose is 8.2 mmol/l. Transvaginal ultrasound demonstrates >10 subcapsular follicles on her ovary, ranging from 2–5 mm in diameter.

(Q140)   A 45-year-old woman presents with weight gain, oligomenorrhoea, galactorrhoea, headaches and visual disturbances, as well as nausea and vomiting. On examination there is mild papilloedema.

Q29

Options:

A   Cabergoline
B   Cyproterone acetate and ethinylestradiol
C   Spironolactone
D   Flutamide
E   Finasteride
F   Eflornithine
G   Norethisterone
H   Danazol
I   Biguanide
J   Clomiphene citrate
K   Ethinylestradiol
L   Estradiol valerate

Lead-in:

For each of the following patients, please select *the most appropriate drug* from the option list. Each option may be used once, more than once, or not at all.

Q141 A 33-year-old parous woman with a BMI of 23 presents with a two-year history of secondary amenorrhoea. Prior to their cessation her periods were regular, and she attributed the changes to stress. There is no galactorrhoea. Clinical examination is normal. A hormone profile reveals the following: FSH 7.9 iU/ml (1–20), LH 9.1 iU/ml (1–20), TSH 4.5 mU/l (0.3–4), prolactin 2650 mU/l (50–500).

Q142 A 28-year-old nulliparous woman with a BMI of 32 presents with a two-year history of oligomenorrhoea. Her periods were irregular since menarche at the age of 13 years, and she was therefore commenced on the COCP when she was 16. She stopped the pill two years ago but her periods have been very infrequent since, only occurring every 3–4 months and lasting 1–2 days. Her LMP was three weeks ago. There is no galactorrhoea or hirsutism. Clinical examination is normal. A hormone profile reveals the following: FSH 4.9 iU/ml (1–20), LH 13.1 iU/ml (1–20), TSH 4.5 mU/l (0.3–4), prolactin 499 mU/l (50–500). Her fasting glucose is 5.8 mmol/l fasting, whilst the two-hour postprandial value is 8.1 mmol/l.

Q143 A 33-year-old nulliparous woman with a BMI of 24 presents with a four-year history of increased facial hair growth, which is causing her considerable distress. She has tried a variety of cosmetic measures, including depilation and laser treatment, with variable success. Her cycles are regular at 4/28. Abdominal and vaginal examination is unremarkable. Transvaginal ultrasound scan confirms a normal pelvis. A hormone profile reveals the following: FSH 3.5 mU/l (1–20), LH 4.2 mU/l (1–20) and FAI 3.5 (2–9).

(Q144) A 25-year-old parous woman with a BMI of 33 is referred to the gynaecology clinic because of oligomenorrhoea and increased facial hair growth. She achieved her only pregnancy after ovulation induction, and had a NVD eight months ago. She breast-fed for six weeks, and had one period at three months postpartum, but no periods since; there is no galactorrhoea. She has no immediate plans for another pregnancy. A hormone profile reveals the following: FSH 3.5 iU/ml (1–20), LH 10.1 iU/ml (1–20), and prolactin 500 mmol/l (50–500).

(Q145) A 29-year-old parous woman with a BMI of 32 is referred to the gynaecology clinic with infrequent periods. She is keen to start a family. Her menarche was at the age of 14; her periods were initially regular but became infrequent eight years ago, following a complete miscarriage at 12 weeks' gestation. Now her periods are up to four months apart, and she bleeds for up to seven days. Her LMP was three weeks ago. There is no galactorrhoea or hirsutism. Clinical examination is normal. A hormone profile reveals the following: FSH 4.9 iU/ml (1–20), LH 5.1 iU/ml (1–20), TSH 3.5 mU/l (0.3–4), prolactin 500 mmol/l (50–500). Transvaginal ultrasound was normal.

Q30

Options:

A   IUI
B   Clomiphene citrate
C   Expectant management
D   Ethinylestradiol
E   Follitropin
F   Medroxyprogesterone acetate
G   Lutropin
H   Human menopausal gonadotrophin

I   IVF
J   ICSI

Lead-in:

For each of the following patients with infertility, please select *the most appropriate management* from the option list. Each option may be used once, more than once, or not at all.

(Q146) A 32-year-old nulliparous woman with a BMI of 28 presents with a nine-month history of amenorrhoea. She is trying for a pregnancy. A hormone profile is reported as: estradiol 70 pmol/l (150–1500), FSH 12 mU/ml (1–20), LH 16 mU/ml (1–20), prolactin 286 mU/l (50–500).

(Q147) A 26-year-old woman with a BMI of 25 presents with amenorrhoea. She has not had a period since she stopped the COCP three months previously and is concerned about her ability to conceive. There is no galactorrhoea, weight gain or hirsutism. A hormone profile is reported as: estradiol <70 pmol/l (150–1500), FSH 4 mU/ml (1–20), LH 7 mU/ml (1–20) and prolactin 157 mU/l (50–500). Semen analysis was declined.

(Q148) A 30-year-old woman with a BMI of 21 presents with a two-year history of primary infertility. She gives a history of regular cycles. She has kept a temperature chart for six cycles. Over the last three cycles her periods commenced 11 days after the rise in basal body temperature. Three blood samples were taken for serum progesterone between days 5–9 post ovulation, and the summed value was 24 ng/ml. Her partner's semen analysis showed a sperm count of 35 million/ml, 88% motile sperm and 36% deformity rate. A HSG was normal.

Q149 A 32-year-old woman with a BMI of 32 presents with primary infertility. She has not used contraception for more than three years, and has failed to conceive despite regular intercourse. Her cycles are regular at 4/28. Day 21 progesterone was 35 ng/ml and 42 ng/ml respectively in two consecutive cycles. She underwent a diagnostic laparoscopy and dye perturbation two years ago, which revealed a normal uterus and ovaries, and free spill of dye was observed from both Fallopian tubes. Two small spots of endometriosis seen on the left uterosacral ligament were treated with laser at the time. Her partner's semen analysis demonstrates a sperm count of 26 million/ml, 78% motile sperm and 25% deformity rate.

Q150 A 36-year-old woman presents with a four-year history of primary infertility. Her cycles are regular at 4/28. Day 21 serum progesterone was 35 ng/ml and 42 ng/ml respectively in two consecutive cycles. A diagnostic laparoscopy and dye pertubation is performed, which demonstrates a 2 cm subserous fibroid on the anterior uterine wall. The left Fallopian tube is distorted with adhesions secondary to endometriosis, but is patent to dye. The right Fallopian tube is normal and also patent. Both ovaries are adherent to the corresponding leaf of the broad ligament, and endometriotic nodules are noted on the left uterosacral ligament. Her partner's semen analysis demonstrates a sperm count of 40 million/ml, 80% motile sperm and 20% deformity rate.

Q31

Options:

A   1–2%
B   3–4%
C   5–6%

D 13%
E 20–25%
F 32%
G 40–50%
H 55–85%
I 90%
J 95%

Lead-in:

For each of the following patients with infertility, please select *the most appropriate success rate* from the option list. Each option may be used once, more than once, or not at all.

(Q151) A 30-year-old woman has failed to conceive for three years despite unprotected intercourse. Her pelvis proves normal on laparoscopy and dye perturbation, and her day-21 serum progesterone is 40 pmol/l. Her partner undergoes semen analysis, which reports semen volume of 3 ml, sperm count of 40 million/ml, 0.5 million/ml white cells are present, with 80% motile sperm and 10% deformity rate. She enquires about her chances of successful pregnancy using IVF.

(Q152) A 34-year-old woman and her 38-year-old male partner have been trying for a pregnancy for the last three years. Her only pregnancy six years ago ended in spontaneous miscarriage. She has normal regular cycles and a biphasic basal temperature chart. You request an HSG which confirms normal tubal patency. Her partner's semen analysis is normal. The couple are considering IVF, but are concerned about the likelihood of congenital malformations in the baby.

(Q153) A 40-year-old woman with regular cycles presents with a long history of infertility. She underwent a termination of pregnancy aged 18, but has not achieved another pregnancy since. Diagnostic laparoscopy and dye pertubation reveal endometriosis in the pouch of Douglas and on the left uterosacral ligament. There are endometriotic adhesions affecting both Fallopian tubes and the right ovary. Her partner's semen analysis is normal. She wishes to know the likely success rate of your suggested intervention.

Q154 A 32-year-old woman presents requesting reversal of sterilisation, which was performed three years ago using Filshie clips. She has two children aged six and eight, but is now in a new relationship. Her partner's semen analysis proves normal. You counsel her about the chances of successful reversal.

Q155 A 25-year-old woman whose partner is aged 28 discontinues the COCP to try for a pregnancy. Her periods are regular, and cyclical symptoms suggest ovulation. Neither she nor her partner have any significant medical problems, and both are fit and healthy and of average body build, however her partner will leave the country in six weeks' time and will return in six months. She asks about the chances of conception over one month of unprotected intercourse.

Urogynaecology

Q32

Options:

A   Pelvic floor exercise
B   Oxybutynin
C   Tolterodine
D   Prazosin hydrochloride
E   Duloxetine hydrochloride
F   Distigmine bromide
G   Sacral nerve stimulation
H   Retropubic mid-urethral tape using macropore tape
I   Botulinum toxin injection
J   Anterior repair
K   Urethral bulking agent
L   Bladder distension surgery
M   Colposuspension
N   Marshall-Marchetti-Krantz procedure
O   Stamey suspension
P   Retropubic suspension using millipore tape

Lead-in:

For each of the following cases, please choose *the most appropriate evidence-based treatment* from the option list. Each option may be used once, more than once, or not at all.

Q156   A 34-year-old Para 2 presents with urinary leakage. Her symptoms occur mainly with coughing and sneezing, but there is also a degree of urgency and on occasion urge incontinence. Physical examination is normal, with no demonstrable incontinence. Urinalysis is negative for leukocytes, blood and protein. You request urodynamic investigations; the report suggests that the bladder was filled at 30 ml/minute to 420 ml. First desire to void was at 85 ml, but the bladder went on to fill to 330 ml before a strong urge to void. During the filling phase there were no unprovoked contractions. On coughing there was no detrusor activity, but there was demonstrable leakage. Voiding was completed at a maximum rate of 13 ml/min, and there was 40 ml residual urine in the bladder.

Q157   A 54-year-old woman, who is three years postmenopausal, presents with urinary leakage. She complains of occasional urinary leakage with coughing and sneezing, severe urgency and on occasion urge incontinence. She wakes three times during the night to pass urine. On examination there is mild descent of the anterior vaginal wall, and demonstrable incontinence with coughing. Urinalysis is negative for leukocytes, blood and protein. You request urodynamics investigations; the report suggests that the bladder was filled at 20 ml/minute, first desire to void occurred at 65 ml, but the bladder went on to fill to 460 ml before a strong urge to void. During the filling phase there were some unprovoked detrusor contractions. Voiding was complete at a maximum rate of 20 ml/min, and there was no residual urine in the bladder.

Q158   A 55-year-old woman with a history of depression, who has been on moclobemide for the past seven years, presents with urinary incontinence. On examination she has demonstrable stress incontinence, but no uterovaginal descent. Urodynamic investigations suggest the diagnosis of USI. She does not respond to first-line therapy initiated by the incontinence advisor.

(Q159) A 78-year-old woman complains of urinary incontinence which is severe enough to interfere with her daily activities. There is no evidence of uterovaginal descent or urinary leakage during pelvic examination; however urodynamic studies suggest the diagnosis of an over-active bladder. Despite persevering, she fails to respond to first-line therapy initiated by the incontinence advisor. Her medication includes isosorbide mononitrate and amiodarone.

(Q160) A 55-year-old woman with a BMI of 36 complains of urinary incontinence. Her symptoms are severe and she has to wear incontinence pads at all times. A bladder diary demonstrates normal volume intake of plain water and some fruit juice. She voids every 3–6 hours, with episodes of urinary leakage with coughing, sneezing or lifting. Clinical examination is normal. Urodynamic studies confirm USI with a stable bladder. First-line therapy advised by the urogynaecology specialist nurse provided only partial relief.

See also:

- National Collaborating Centre for Women's and Children's Health. *The Management of Urinary Incontinence in Women.* Commissioned by the National Institute for Health and Clinical Excellence. London: RCOG Press; October 2006.
- Adams EJ, Barrington JW, Brown K, Smith ARB. *Surgical Treatment of Urodynamic Stress Incontinence.* Guideline No. 35. London: Royal College of Obstetricians and Gynaecologists; October 2003.

Gynaecological oncology

Q33

Options:

A Watchful waiting
B External beam radiotherapy
C High-dose progestogens
D Cisplatin and 5-fluorouracil
E External beam radiotherapy + cisplatin
F Paclitaxel + carboplatin
G External beam radiotherapy + paclitaxel
H Anastrazol
I Vaginal brachytherapy
J Methotrexate + paclitaxel

Lead-in:

For each of the patients with gynaecological malignancy described below, please identify *the most effective therapy* from the option list. Each option may be used once, more than once, or not at all.

 A 56-year-old woman undergoes a TAH and BSO for endometrial cancer. No staging lymphadenectomy was performed, but there were no malignant cells in the peritoneal aspirate and no para-aortic lymphadenopathy. The liver was normal, and there was no enlargement of supra-clavicular or inguinal lymph nodes. Histological examination demonstrates invasion of one-third of the myometrium, with involvement of the cervical stroma.

Q162 A 32-year-old woman has been treated by her GP for irregular vaginal bleeding for nine months without success. On referral to gynaecology, a large ulcerated area is noted on the cervix and a biopsy confirms adenosquamous carcinoma G3. Examination under anaesthesia demonstrates a central lesion 4.2 cm in diameter and some thickening to the left cardinal ligament. The upper vagina is disease free. Cystoscopy reveals oedema in the region of the trigone; urine cytology demonstrated leukocytes, but no malignant cells.

Q163 A 63-year-old woman undergoes a TAH and BSO for recurrent postmenopausal bleeding after repeatedly negative endometrial biopsy. During the operation she is noted to have a nodule in the right Fallopian tube of approximately 2 cm in size, raising the suspicion of carcinoma of the Fallopian tube. Peritoneal washings are therefore obtained and omentectomy is carried out. Peritoneal cavity, omentum and liver appear normal. Histological assessment confirms an adenocarcinoma G2, confined to the right Fallopian tube. Peritoneal washings and omentum are negative, as is a CXR.

Q164 A 71-year-old woman presents with increasing abdominal distension and anorexia. Pelvi-abdominal examination is consistent with an ovarian mass and ascites. Chest X-ray is normal. She subsequently undergoes a midline laparotomy and is noted to have a friable tumour arising from her right ovary; the left ovary is normal. There are visible nodules on the omentum, two nodules (1 cm in diameter) are noted on the diaphragm and para-aortic lymph nodes are enlarged. Malignancy is confirmed on histological examination of the pelvic, but not the para-aortic, nodes. Peritoneal and omental biopsies confirm G3 mucinous carcinoma.

A 73-year-old woman undergoes *en bloc* vulvectomy with bilateral inguinofemoral lymphadenectomy for carcinoma of the vulva. Histology reports a 1.5 cm well-differentiated squamous carcinoma of the vulva. One ipsilateral lymph node was positive for tumour involvement of 3 mm.

Q34

Options:

A   Stage Ia
B   Stage Ib
C   Stage Ic
D   Stage IIa
E   Stage IIb
F   Stage IIc
G   Stage IIIa
H   Stage IIIb
I   Stage IIIc
J   Stage IVa
K   Stage IVb

Lead-in:

For each of the following cases of gynaecological cancer, please select *the correct FIGO stage* from the option list. Each option may be used once, more than once, or not at all.

 A 56-year-old woman undergoes a TAH and BSO for endometrial cancer. Histological examination demonstrated invasion of one-third of the myometrium, with involvement of the cervical stroma. No staging lymphadenectomy was performed, but there were no malignant cells in the peritoneal aspirate and no para-aortic lymphadenopathy.

The liver was normal, and there was no enlargement of supraclavicular or inguinal lymph nodes.

(Q167) A 32-year-old woman has been treated by her GP for irregular vaginal bleeding for nine months without success. When she presented to gynaecology, a larger ulcerating area was noted to replace the cervix. Biopsy proved cervical adenosquamous carcinoma G3. Examination under anaesthesia demonstrates a central lesion 4.2 cm in diameter and some thickening to the left cardinal ligament. The upper vagina is disease free. Cystoscopy reveals oedema in the region of the trigone; urine cytology demonstrated leukocytes, but no malignant cells.

(Q168) A 63-year-old woman undergoes a TAH and BSO for recurrent postmenopausal bleeding after repeatedly negative endometrial biopsy. During the operation she is noted to have a nodule in the right Fallopian tube of approximately 2 cm in size. Peritoneal washings are therefore obtained and omentectomy is carried out. Peritoneal cavity, omentum and liver appear normal. Histological assessment confirms an adeno-carcinoma G2, confined to the right Fallopian tube. Peritoneal washings and omentum are negative, as is a CXR.

(Q169) A 71-year-old woman presents with increasing abdominal distension and anorexia. Pelvi-abdominal examination is consistent with an ovarian mass and ascites. Chest X-ray is normal. She subsequently undergoes a midline laparotomy and is noted to have a friable tumour arising from her right ovary; the left ovary is normal. There are visible nodules on the omentum, two nodules (1 cm in diameter) are noted on the diaphragm and para-aortic lymph nodes are enlarged. Malignancy is confirmed on histological examination of the pelvic, but not the para-aortic, nodes. Peritoneal and omental biopsies confirm G3 mucinous carcinoma.

(Q170) A 70-year-old woman with a long-standing history of lichen sclerosus et atrophicus presents with a new pruritic vulval lesion. On examination there is an ulcerated lesion of approximately 1.5 cm diameter on the left labium majus, with multiple surrounding excoriations. The lesion is sampled, and histopathology suggests a squamous cell carcinoma with maximum depth of invasion of 0.8 mm.

Therapeutics in obstetrics and gynaecology

Q35

Options:

A Estradiol valerate + levonorgestrel
B Ethinylestradiol + cyproterone acetate
C Ethinylestradiol + norelgestromin
D Gestrinone
E Etonogestrel
F Ethynodiol diacetate
G Megesterol acetate
H Ethinylestradiol + desogestrel
I Ethinylestradiol + drospirenone
J Ethinylestradiol + levonorgestrel

Lead in:

For each of the patients requiring medication described below, please recommend *the most suitable sex steroid combination* from the option list. Each option may be used once, more than once, or not at all.

(Q171) A 24-year-old university student with insulin-dependent diabetes is seeking a reliable contraceptive with good cycle control. She is a nulliparous non-smoker with a BMI of 22 and her cycles are regular at 4/28, but she occasionally has mid-cycle bleeding. Her diabetes is uncomplicated and well controlled, and she leads an active lifestyle. There is no significant family history of medical problems.

(Q172) An 18-year-old woman, who is not in a stable relationship currently, is seeking a reliable contraceptive. She has a history of an ectopic pregnancy and a recent surgical termination of pregnancy. She has just completed a drug rehabilitation programme, and is known to miss hospital and clinic appointments frequently.

(Q173) A 34-year-old woman has given birth to a healthy baby girl. She has been on the COCP in the past without problems, but intends to breast-feed her baby.

(Q174) A 36-year-old Asian woman presents seeking contraceptive advice; she has a strong family history of hypertension and heart disease. Her blood pressure has been borderline, and her BMI is 30. Her periods are regular but heavy, and on examination you find the uterus to be enlarged to 12 weeks' size with fibroids. She tells you that she has been using condoms for the last year, but these have been unsatisfactory.

(Q175) A 28-year-old woman presents with severe dysmenorrhoea and deep dyspareunia. Her cycles are regular. Diagnostic laparoscopy reveals pelvic endometriosis. She has endometriotic nodules in the POD and related adhesions around the left ovary. She gives a history of raised BP on the COCP and is currently using condoms for contraception.

Q36

Options:

A   Levonorgestrel
B   Progesterone
C   Medroxyprogesterone acetate
D   Drospirenone
E   Ethynodiol diacetate
F   Cyproterone acetate
G   Etonogestrel
H   Norelgestromin
I   Norethynodrel
J   Dydrogesterone

Lead-in:

For each of the patients described below, please choose *the most appropriate progestogen* from the option list. Each option may be used once, more than once, or not at all.

 A 24-year-old woman presents to the family planning clinic on day 16 of her current cycle, having had unprotected intercourse on days 13 and 14. She is nulliparous and her cycles are regular at 4/28.

 A 26-year-old mother of twins presents for contraceptive advice. She has been on the same COCP for two years, but recently noted increased breast discomfort and break-through bleeding during most of her cycles.

 A 23-year-old nulliparous woman attends her GP's surgery for contraceptive advice. She is about to join an aid agency and will be posted to a developing country with poor access to medical services for the coming 12 months, and is unlikely to be planning for a pregnancy for a number of years. She would like a long-acting, reversible method of contraception.

Q179   A 34-year-old nulliparous woman asks you for contraceptive advice; her periods are light and infrequent, she has a BMI of 30 kg/m^2. She also complains of increased facial hair and acne.

Q180   A 36-year-old mother of two presents seeking contraceptive advice. Her periods are regular and average, she is of average build and has no significant past medical history. She has used the COCP successfully for the last four years, but because of the 'school run' is worried about missing her pill. She does not favour long-acting preparations or those likely to alter her menstrual cycle.

Q37

Options:

A   Retinol
B   Cobalamine
C   Ascorbic acid
D   Cholecalciferol
E   Folic acid
F   Thiamin
G   Phytomenadione
H   Niacin
I   Folinic acid
J   Pyridoxine

Lead-in:

For each of the case scenarios described below, please select *the most relevant substance* from the option list. Each option may be used once, more than once, or not at all.

 A 59-year-old postmenopausal woman consults her GP regarding her family history of osteoporosis.

 A 29-year-old woman is receiving treatment for chorio-carcinoma following a molar pregnancy. She develops a sore mouth.

 A 30-year-old woman is planning to start a family. She has a family history of neural tube defects.

 A 19-year-old primigravida has been hospitalised with hyperemesis gravidarum. She has been unable to eat or drink for 10 days now, and her liver function tests are mildly deranged.

 A 33-year-old woman is seen at 32 weeks' gestation with generalised pruritus without a rash.

Audit, research and management

Q38

Options:

A Lead time bias
B Length time bias
C Screening bias
D Recall bias
E Selection bias
F Publication bias
G Assessment bias
H Response bias
I Type 2 error
J Skewness

Lead-in:

For each of the scenarios, please select *the most likely statistical problem* from the option list. Each option may be used once, more than once, or not at all.

 A randomised controlled trial is conducted to compare two doses of mifepristone for induction of labour. Women with a uterine scar, IUGR, diabetes or pre-eclampsia are excluded. All women admitted for IOL are approached, but the uptake is lower amongst women from ethnic minority groups.

(Q187) A study is conducted to assess the reliability of cervical smear testing. All women who over the previous two years had a recall because of inadequate or borderline smear report had their smear re-examined by a different histopathologist. There was disagreement between the two assessors in four out of the 200 cases examined. It was concluded that the accuracy of cervical smear reporting by the laboratory is 98%.

(Q188) A randomised controlled study is conducted to compare the outcome of TVT versus duloxetine in women with urinary stress incontinence. After six months women were asked to prospectively complete a bladder diary over one week.

(Q189) A cervical screening programme is set up in a deprived area. The uptake of screening is around 75–85%, and the detected incidence of CIN is low. The incidence of CIN III in the catchment area is within the national average.

(Q190) A study is set up to assess risk factors for cervical cancer. At enrolment, patients are asked to complete a questionnaire detailing age at menarche, past use of the pill, as well as menstrual and sexual history.

Q39

Options:

A Analysis of variance
B Paired student t-test
C Unpaired student t-test
D Receiver operating characteristic curves (ROC)
E Wilcoxon signed rank test

F   Mann-Whitney U
G   Multiple regression
H   Chi-squared test
I   Fisher's exact test
J   Meta-analysis
K   Correlation coefficient
L   Kappa coefficient
M   Kaplan-Meier survival curve
N   Hazard ratio

Lead-in:

For each of the following scenarios, please select *the most appropriate statistical descriptor* from the option list. Each option may be used once, more than once, or not at all.

Q191   In a published study, 33/90 (37%) women with previous tubal sterilisation, and 19/84 (23%) women without tubal sterilisation, reported pain and/or dysmenorrhoea following roller-ball endometrial ablation. Nineteen (21%) women with previous sterilisation, and four (5%) women without tubal sterilisation, reported new or worsening pain.

Q192   A questionnaire study compared women's experience of giving written consent to elective or emergency surgery. Of those undergoing elective surgery, 80% were satisfied, 16% were neither satisfied or dissatisfied, and 4% were dissatisfied/very dissatisfied. The corresponding figures for women undergoing emergency surgery were 63% , 30%, and 7% respectively.

Q193   In a questionnaire study comparing women's experience of giving written consent to elective or emergency surgery, a total of 734 questionnaires were returned, giving a response rate of 71%. Non-responders were likely to be younger (mean age 36.9 vs. 39.8) than responders.

Q194 A retrospective postal questionnaire study was undertaken to examine the outcomes of endometrial ablation using 'Cavaterm *plus*'. The mean follow-up postoperatively was 72 weeks. A total of 103 patients completed the questionnaire; 19.4% women had procedure-related amenorrhoea, 10.7% had subsequently had a hysterectomy. The risk of failure was inversely related to age (OR 0.78, 95% CI 0.69–0.95) and was higher in women who prior to surgery had longer duration of bleeding problems (OR 1.29, 95% CI 1.1–1.52).

Q195 A study was conducted to assess the long-term effectiveness of endometrial laser ablation. Postal questionnaires were sent to all women who underwent endometrial laser ablation 1.5–9 years previously. A total of 174 patients returned the questionnaire. The procedure was reported as a success by 79.3% and a failure by 21%. Twenty-four patients (13.8%) subsequently underwent hysterectomy for excessive bleeding. At one year, 95.3% procedures were reported as successful, but this dropped to 76.2% at four years.

Q40

Options:

A   Cost-effectiveness analysis
B   Opportunity cost
C   Cost-utility analysis
D   Quality-adjusted life years
E   Health utility
F   Cost-benefit analysis
G   Discounting
H   Conjoint analysis
I   Cost-minimisation analysis
J   Cost function

Lead-in:

For each of the health economic issues below, please select *the most appropriate methodology* from the option list. Each option may be used once, more than once, or not at all.

 Both radiotherapy and radical surgery are recognised treatments for women with stage Ia cervical cancer. Consideration was given to compare both treatment modalities when setting up a new service at a tertiary treatment centre with reference to post-treatment survival.

 A researcher set out to compare the use of the MEA technique in outpatient and day-case settings. The outcomes of both groups turned out to be equivalent.

 You are setting up a high-risk pregnancy service for women with endocrine problems. You wish to consider routine screening for gestational diabetes against selective testing in women based on identified risk factors.

 A gynaecology department acquires new funds. Decisions have to be made as to whether these should be spent on an improved palliative care service for women with ovarian cancer or a new diagnostic service for women with infertility. The views of the local users were sought, including their willingness to pay for both types of services. This was entered into the calculation of likely benefit of the services.

Hysterectomy and endometrial ablation for the treatment of heavy regular periods are compared. Eighteen percent of women undergoing endometrial ablation had a recurrence of symptoms over four years of follow-up. This resulted in fewer disease-free years compared to hysterectomy.

Ethics and law in obstetrics and gynaecology

Q41

Options:

A Confidentiality
B Fraser (Gillick) competence
C Non-maleficence
D Negligence
E Paternalism
F Fidelity
G Veracity
H Battery
I Beneficence
J Bolam test
K Autonomy

Lead-in:

For each of the following scenarios, please select *the most applicable medico-legal principle* from the option list. Each option can be used once, more than once, or not at all.

(Q201) A 29-year-old primigravida is admitted to the labour ward at 25/40 gestation in what appears to be advanced labour. She is very distressed and communication is difficult. Within 20 minutes of admission she delivers a live male infant, and a neonatologist is crash-bleeped. The patient screams at the doctor to leave the baby alone and to not resuscitate him.

(Q202) A 30-year-old G3 P2, who has had two previous uncomplicated vaginal deliveries, goes into labour at 38 weeks' gestation. Because of delay in the first stage, labour is augmented with oxytocin. The patient progresses to full cervical dilatation, but remains undelivered after two hours in the second stage. The doctor on duty is called to review her and documents the following: cervix is fully dilated, DOA at spines, 0/5 palpable abdominally. A decision is made to proceed with instrumental delivery. The vacuum extraction fails after the cup detaches twice, and delivery is achieved using a Neville-Barnes forceps. The head delivers in occipitoposterior position and a shoulder dystocia follows; the baby is delivered by Wood's Screw manoeuvre as the McRoberts' manoeuvre and suprapubic pressure are unsuccessful. The baby is noted to have Erb's palsy.

(Q203) During an audit, your hospital laboratory uncovered an error in labelling of a number of cervical smear specimens dated back to 1995–1998. A high-level urgent meeting is called to discuss whether disclosure is in the best interest of the trust.

(Q204) A 50-year-old woman with learning difficulties is admitted with postmenopausal bleeding, which seems to have been ongoing for a number of weeks. Communication is difficult, but she seems to be refusing to have any investigations done. Her carer wants her to undergo investigations to ascertain the cause of bleeding.

Q205 An 18-year-old primigravida with poor command of English attends the antenatal clinic with her 36-year-old husband, who always acts as an interpreter. At 36 weeks' gestation you note that the baby is in breech presentation. An ultrasound scan suggests oligohydramnios. You recommend a Caesarean section, but the husband refuses to translate this recommendation to his wife. The patient does not express an opinion herself. When you try to explain the risks of vaginal breech delivery, the husband leaves the room and she follows.

Q42

Options:

A   Offences Against the Person Act 1861
B   Human Tissue Act 2004
C   European Convention on Human Rights, Articles 8 and 9
D   European Convention on Human Rights, Articles 1 and 2
E   Mental Health Act 1983
F   Data Protection Act 1998
G   Abortion Act 1967
H   Anatomy Act 1984
I   Freedom of Information Act 2000
J   National Health Service (Primary Care) Act 1997

Lead-in:

For each case scenario described below, please select *the applicable legal framework* from the option list. Each option may be used once, more than once, or not at all.

A 23-year-old woman, who lives in a remote rural area, attends her local GP practice requesting a termination of pregnancy. Her GP is on leave and the only available doctor is strongly anti-abortion.

Q207 A 70-year-old woman is admitted to hospital for a laparotomy because of a pelvic mass, presumed to be ovarian in origin. Her family request to speak to you, and ask you not to disclose the diagnosis to the patient if the tumour is malignant because of their concerns for her psychological well-being.

Q208 A 30-year-old primigravida has a placenta praevia. She is scheduled to undergo an elective Caesarean section at 39 weeks' gestation. She informs you that she is a Jehovah's Witness and that she will not accept a blood transfusion under any circumstances. During the Caesarean section she develops a massive haemorrhage and dies.

Q209 A 21-year-old woman who suffers with schizophrenia attends hospital. She is distressed to find herself eight weeks pregnant. Her mental illness has been difficult to control, and she lives in a residential mental healthcare facility. Her carer suggests that a TOP would be in her best interest. She seems to concur.

Q210 Your hospital pathology laboratory plans an audit involving all cervical biopsies obtained over the previous year for the purpose of quality control.

ANSWERS

Applied basic sciences

Q1

(A1) A. The likely mechanism here is Müllerian agenesis as the patient has a normal female phenotype and normal ovaries, but a uterus was not visualised during a pelvic ultrasound.

(A2) E. The fact that the doctor can only identify one tube suggests a unicornuate uterus. In a markedly dextro-rotated uterus, the left Fallopian tube would be anterior, and we can therefore assume that it is the right-sided paramesonephric duct that has not developed here.

(A3) C. This is a uterus didelphis, so the Müllerian ducts have failed to fuse.

(A4) F. This is an imperforate hymen, with a failure of the Müllerian system and the sinovaginal bulb to complete their connection.

(A5) D. This patient has a septate uterus. The paramesonephric ducts have fused here, as she has a single uterus which is not bicornuate, but the septum has not been fully broken down.

Q2

(A6) **B.** Uterine artery embolisation is a recognised treatment for uterine fibroids in women wishing to conserve their uterus or avoid surgery. A systematic review in 2004 found that fibroids shrank in approximately 60% and some symptom relief was reported in >90% of patients. Complication rates were at least similar to those with hysterectomy, and up to 14% of patients were reported to have developed ovarian dysfunction, ranging from irregular menstruation to ovarian failure. (See also www.nice.org.uk/download.aspx?o=ip020 systematicreview.)

(A7) **I.** Sacrospinous fixation is the procedure referred to in this scenario, which is of course performed vaginally.

(A8) **M.** This scenario describes an obturator nerve injury. The anterior rami of L2, L3 and L4 fuse to form this nerve within the psoas muscle and emerge laterally to the sacrum under the common iliac vessels. The obturator nerve then courses through the obturator foramen and enters the thigh. The motor branches supply the adductor brevis, adductor longus and gracilis muscles. Obturator nerve injury can lead to abnormal gait with an external rotation of the foot.

(A9) **P.** Ureteric injury is less common in gynaecological surgery than bladder or bowel injury; however, it has a high morbidity with fistula formation and potential loss of renal function. Typical injury to the ureter may include ligation, angulation with secondary obstruction, transection, thermal injury/ischaemia and crush injury from incorrectly applied clamps. Most ureteric injuries occur at the site of its proximity to the cervix, although it is also at risk near the infundibulopelvic ligament where the abdominal approach is used.

(A10) **N.** The inferior epigastric artery, a branch of the external iliac artery, is at risk during laparoscopic entry in the abdomen. It has been suggested that lateral ports should be placed at least 8 cm from the midline and 5 cm above the symphysis pubis to avoid vascular injury.

Q3

(A11) G. This patient presents with a probable iliofemoral venous thrombosis. DVT is only confirmed in around 50% of patients with classic signs; these include pain and tenderness in the limb and along the affected vein and swelling of calf or thigh. Involvement of the iliac bifurcation, pelvic veins or vena cava results in leg oedema. The superficial veins may appear distended, and there may be increased skin temperature, skin discolouration, erythema or pallor.

(A12) E. The case history is suggestive of a ureteric/renal colic. Renal pain usually presents as a dull ache in the costo-vertebral angle and upper outer quadrant of the abdomen. Pain passing from the loin to the groin is typical of ureteric colic.

(A13) E. Cervical fibroids form about 5% of all fibroids. With few exceptions cervical fibroids tend to displace the uterine arteries upwards, and the ureter outwards. The ureters can become obstructed, causing hydronephrosis.

(A14) J. Pudendal block involves the administration of local anaesthetic around the pudendal nerve as it passes behind the sacrospinous ligament. Complications include intravascular injection, haematoma and, rarely, infection in the region of the gluteal muscles. The internal pudendal artery is a branch of the posterior division of the internal iliac artery. It descends anterior to piriformis muscle and the sacral plexus, leaves the pelvis through the greater sciatic foramen passing over the posterior surface of the ischial spine, and enters the perineum through the lesser sciatic foramen.

(A15) B. The femoral nerve arises from the dorsal division of L2–4 and emerges from the psoas muscle below the iliac crest to enter the thigh lateral to the femoral sheath. The femoral nerve innervates the quadriceps muscle and carries sensory nerves from the anterior aspect of the thigh and medial leg and foot. Patients with femoral neuropathy complain of difficulty walking stairs and frequent falling secondary to 'knee buckling'. Sensory symptoms include tingling and numbness along the sensory distribution. Femoral nerve injury is the most commonly encountered nerve injury in gynaecological surgery. Risk factors include wide transverse incisions, BMI <20, prolonged surgery and deep retractor blades.

Q4

(A16) C. The examination findings suggest a well-flexed head, which means that the structure with the most relevant dimension here will be the suboccipitobregmatic circumference. As the presenting part is below the ischial spines, the interspinous diameter has already been navigated.

(A17) E. The findings here indicate a vertex presentation in occipitoposterior position, implying a degree of deflection; the structure with the most relevant dimension to the progress of labour here will be the occipitofrontal circumference. A grand multipara, who has had previous uncomplicated vaginal deliveries, is unlikely to have suboptimal pelvic diameters, and the malposition is likely to be the key element here.

(A18) A. This clinical scenario suggests a contracted pelvic inlet. The examination findings describe the diagonal conjugate, the only inlet diameter that can be assessed directly during vaginal examination. The obstetric conjugate can only be estimated indirectly from the diagonal conjugate, by subtracting 1.5 cm.

(A19) F. This is a mentoposterior face presentation; the structure with the most relevant dimension here will be the submentobregmatic circumference. The mentovertical circumference presents in a brow presentation, where a lesser degree of extension is present.

(A20) J. This is a vertex presentation with a 'military' (or neutral) attitude, as both fontanelles can be palpated. The structure with the most relevant dimension here will be the suboccipitofrontal circumference.

Q5

(A21) A. The mitochondrial genome is a circular DNA molecule that encodes rRNA, tRNA and part of the polypeptide chains of the oxidative phosphorylation system. The ovum is the source of all mitochondria in the embryo, as mitochondria contained in the sperm is located in the tail region which does not penetrate the ovum at fertilisation. No known disease is believed to be inherited through paternal mitochondria. It is probable that mitochondrial mutation is involved in a small proportion of cases of NIDDM.

(A22) C. This describes the mechanism of genomic imprinting. Genomic imprinting refers to the process by which specific genes are marked during parental gametogenesis, resulting in differential expression of these genes depending on their origin (paternal or maternal). Genomic imprinting is thought to be relevant to X-chromosome inactivation, and is thought to play a role in diseases such as Prader-Willi and Angelman syndrome.

(A23) E. This child appears to have Prader-Willi syndrome (PWS). Affected individuals have short stature, dysmorphic features, obesity, polyphagia, hypogonadism and mental retardation. PWS results from uniparental disomy, where both copies of a gene are inherited from the same parent; in this case both copies of chromosome 15 are inherited from the mother. Other conditions thought to be associated with uniparental disomy include Beckwith-Wiedeman and Angelman syndrome. The sequelae of uniparental disomy are largely the result of genomic imprinting.

(A24) B. About three-quarters of the genome consists of unique DNA, the remainder consists of several classes of tandem repeats that vary in length. Expansion of trinucleotide repeat sequences is now recognised as a cause of a number of human diseases such as fragile X syndrome and Huntington's disease. Fragile X affects 1:1200 males and 1:2500 females. Approximately 1:700 females will carry the fragile X mutation (*FMR-1*) gene.

(A25) B. The family history is suggestive of Huntington's disease; the mode of inheritance is autosomal dominant. The affected gene on the short arm of chromosome 4 contains an expanded and unstable triple trinucleotide repeat.

Q6

(A26) G. The inheritance trait is recessive.

(A27) C. The overall recurrence risk for trisomy 21 is 1%.

(A28) B. The inheritance trait is autosomal dominant.

(A29) E. The recurrence risk of NTD is approximately 1:20, although there are figures suggesting a range or risk from 2–5%. The incidence of NTD varies, depending on population studied, from 1:2500 to 1:100 live births (worldwide average of 1:500), and recurrence risk is likely to be subject to similar differences. Additionally, the incidence of NTD seems to go through peaks and troughs; overall, the incidence is falling – this is not thought to be simply a reflection of prenatal screening and termination of pregnancy, but a multifactorial development.

A30 E. The risk of congenital heart disease in the offspring of affected individuals is approximately 5%, although some differences exist depending on the type of defect.

Reproductive health

Q7

(A31) B. You will be aware that typical use carries a higher failure rate than ideal use, particularly in methods which depend on patient compliance. With COCP failure will occur with missed pills, enzyme-inducing drugs, and gastrointestinal disturbances.

(A32) E. Partly due to lost or poorly placed device, although a proportion will be genuine method failures.

(A33) F. The failures following female sterilisation may be the result of incorrect application technique (occlusion of wrong structure, incomplete occlusion), pre-existing pregnancy or recanalisation.

(A34) G. It is worth remembering that withdrawal is better than no contraception at all!

(A35) I. Condom failures are often associated with poor application technique, slippage, breakage, or the use of incorrect lubricant.

Q8

(A36) F. The risk of venous thromboembolism with third-generation COCP is approximately 1:5000, which is about double of that quoted for COCP users overall.

(A37) B. The risk of venous thromboembolism in thrombophilia carriers is substantially higher than the risk in individuals without thrombogenic mutations.

(A38) D. The risk of perforation during IUCD insertion is approximately 1:1000.

(A39) H. The POP is not associated with a significant increase in the risk of thrombosis, therefore the background risk will apply. However, it is worth remembering that the increased risk of thrombosis observed with third-generation COCP was largely related to the type of progestogen used – there was a two to threefold increased risk among users of third-generation oral contraceptives containing the progestogen desogestrel and gestodene. The quoted thrombosis incidence rates per 100,000 woman-years among COCP users are 16.1 for levonorgestrel users, 29.3 for desogestrel and 28.1 for gestodene. (See also www.rila.co.uk/issues/full/download/142ac447c05bf1ec 0378eaf96c386eb9702524.pdf.)

(A40) J. The mortality from legal termination of pregnancy is in the region of 0.4 in 100,000. In the Confidential Inquiry into Maternal Deaths for the 2000–2002 triennium, there were five deaths related to termination of pregnancy; causes included sepsis, pulmonary embolism, anaesthetic complications, and deaths related to pre-existing risk factors such as morbid obesity and cardiac disease (see www.cemach.org.uk/publications/WMD2000_2002/wmd-06.htm).

Q9

The following questions will be easy to answer for those who have looked at the RCOG Green Top Guideline on Acute Pelvic Inflammatory Disease at www.rcog.org.uk/resources/Public/pdf/Pelvic_Inflamatory_Disease_No32.pdf.

(A41)   D. Mild to moderate PID can be managed in the community, with hospital referral if first-line management fails or if the patient's condition deteriorates. Treatment should be started as soon as the condition is suspected. First-line treatment would be ofloxacin and metronidazole orally, for a full 14 days. Alternatively, a stat dose of intramuscular ceftriaxone and oral probenecid can be administered, followed by a 14-day course of oral metronidazole and doxycycline.

(A42)   D. The scenario here is similar to the one above and requires the same treatment regimen. The complicating factor here is that conception may have occurred in this cycle. Administration of the appropriate antibiotics in very early pregnancy is likely to result in an 'all or nothing' scenario rather than teratogenicity. PID from the late first trimester onward is very rare.

(A43)   H. In severe PID intravenous therapy is required; again, the combination of ofloxacin and metronidazole may be used, for a 14-day period. Alternatives include intravenous clindamycin and gentamicin, followed by oral doxycycline and metronidazole, or intravenous cefoxitine, followed by oral doxycycline and metronidazole.

(A44)   H. Failure to respond to first-line oral therapy is an indication for intravenous treatment.

(A45)   D. The IUCD may be left *in situ* initially, and oral treatment commenced as per usual. Removal of the IUCD may need to be considered where the patient fails to respond to first-line treatment.

Q10

(A46) I. This patient clearly has significant mental illness, which required hospitalisation. Additionally, the history suggests a difficulty in finding effective therapy; the tricyclic anti-depressant she is on appears to be effective, and it would therefore be counterproductive to discontinue it at this point. Data on use in pregnancy is limited, however there is no convincing evidence of teratogenicity and routine discontinuation in pregnancy is not recommended. (See also www.sign.ac.uk/guidelines/fulltext/60/section4.html.) Breast-feeding is possible with tricyclics, with the exception of doxepine. As with most obstetric patients with a chronic illness, the relevant specialist should be consulted before medication is changed or discontinued.

(A47) H. You should be able to answer this question even if you have not heard of bosentan! This patient's history suggests that she might have pulmonary hypertension, which has a high maternal mortality. Without discussion with the patient's cardiologist, it would be unwise to advise pregnancy. Bosentan is a vasodilator used in the treatment of pulmonary hypertension, and is teratogenic.

(A48) D. This patient may have had severe reactive depression following the tragic death of her family. As the events, including her inpatient treatment, are fairly recent, it is reasonable to assume that treatment should be continued. You will be aware that paroxetine is an SSRI. In general, there is no need to routinely withdraw SSRIs in pregnancy; however, paroxetine is the SSRI with the most controversial safety profile. Recent data suggest an increased risk of congenital malformations, including omphalocele, cranio-synostosis and congenital heart defects with its use in the first trimester, and neonatal withdrawal symptoms also seem to be most pronounced with paroxetine. Whilst the strength of the evidence is under discussion, another SSRI (fluoxetine) should probably be used where it is thought that treatment should be continued in pregnancy.

(A49) E. As this patient has been seizure free for five years, reduction to monotherapy may be considered in discussion with the patient's neurologist. Clearly, the preferred treatment here would be monotherapy with lamotrigine. Ideally, this should be accomplished before conception to allow a period of assessment following changes to medication.

(A50) A. Simvastatin can be reasonably withdrawn here, as it is unlikely that a temporary discontinuation of the treatment will have a significant impact on the patient's long-term outcome. Whilst women should receive appropriate treatment for their medical condition during pregnancy, non-essential medication is best avoided.

Normal and complicated pregnancy

Q11

(A51) B. The serum ßHCG and progesterone levels suggest a failed pregnancy. Because of the time scale, this pregnancy failure would be termed a biochemical pregnancy, i.e. a pregnancy that fails before any sonographic evidence can be expected.

(A52) I. This is most likely to be an ectopic pregnancy which was not diagnosed prior to the medical TOP. The intrauterine mixed echogenic mass may be a blood clot or decidual debris, whilst the adnexal mass may represent the ectopic pregnancy. The differential diagnosis would be a failed/incomplete termination of pregnancy with a corpus luteum, however the clinical scenario dictates that an ectopic pregnancy has to be excluded.

(A53) C. The case scenario here suggests an incomplete miscarriage, with failed attempt at medical evacuation of the uterus.

(A54) E. The route of ultrasound examination is not given in the patient vignette, which makes things somewhat more difficult. However, whilst a viable intrauterine pregnancy remains a possibility, in view of the high ßHCG level for the gestation, a mole has to be a leading differential diagnosis in the absence of a fetal pole. One should, of course, also consider the possibility of an undiagnosed multiple pregnancy.

(A55) **A.** The ßHCG profile suggests an ongoing pregnancy, which is probably earlier in terms of gestation than the period of amenorrhoea implies. The fact that the patient presented with vaginal bleeding would make the diagnosis at this point a threatened miscarriage.

Q12

The candidate should refer to the RCOG Green Top Guideline on Anti-D Policy (see <u>www.rcog.org.uk/index.asp?PageID=512</u>).

 H. Rhesus negative, non-sensitised women undergoing TOP before 20 weeks' gestation should be given 250 iU of anti-D immunoglobulin.

(A57) **G.** Postnatally, an estimation of fetomaternal haemorrhage should be made to identify those women who require a larger dose of anti-D immunoglobulin than administered routinely (500 iU in the UK). The presence of anti-Kell has no impact on the rhesus status management.

 H. All non-sensitised women who are rhesus negative should receive anti-D immunoglobulin following an ectopic pregnancy.

(A59) **G.** A dose of at least 500 iU of anti-D immunoglobulin is required to cover potentially sensitising events after 20 weeks' gestation, but fetomaternal haemorrhage should always be quantified to identify women requiring an additional dose to 'mop up' the bleed.

(A60) **D.** Most women who are Jehovah's Witness will decline human (non-recombinant) blood products; this often applies to anti-D immunoglobulin. It is not uncommon for these patients to request partner testing to establish the need for prophylaxis. In this case, both the parents are rhesus negative. However, one should bear in mind that in a proportion of couples, paternity may be unclear or undisclosed. It is worth noting that this patient may be at risk of developing anti-E antibodies, and atypical antibody screening should be carried out in the recommended fashion.

Q13

(A61) L. Uterine artery Doppler is a screening test for pre-eclampsia and severe early-onset IUGR; however, its value in a low-risk population is limited and current evidence only supports its use in high-risk women. The positive predictive value is low, but the negative predictive value at 24/40 gestation is >90%.

(A62) E. The value of a GTT after 32–34 weeks' gestation is limited; however, an HbA1c will provide information on blood sugar levels over the preceding six weeks.

(A63) K. Recurrent confirmed UTIs require a renal ultrasound to exclude underlying renal problems such as hydronephrosis.

(A64) H. Glycosuria in the first trimester should be investigated, as a proportion of these patients may have undiagnosed diabetes; the most appropriate test is an oral GTT.

(A65) I. The patient is normotensive and asymptomatic at presentation. The only positive finding is + of proteinuria on urinalysis. Aside from a clinical assessment, a urinary protein–creatinine ratio will help quantify the proteinuria. Whilst an isolated episode of + of proteinuria is not usually a cause for concern, in view of previous pre-eclampsia it may be reasonable to get a baseline measurement.

Q14

(A66) K. This patient appears to have presented with significant symptoms of imminent eclampsia. The most appropriate initial management would be seizure prophylaxis using magnesium sulphate, whilst a full assessment of her condition is being made.

(A67) G. At 29 weeks' gestation, one would wish to temporise to avoid extreme prematurity, provided it is safe to do so. Again, a comprehensive assessment of the maternal condition should be made. It is reasonable to quantify the proteinuria to allow monitoring of disease progression in due course. Whilst this patient's blood pressure does not yet warrant treatment, it is likely that she will require anti-hypertensive treatment in the near future.

(A68) D. In the presence of significant hypertension in the first trimester, it is advisable to start oral antihypertensives.

(A69) J. The presence of unilateral abdominal pain and irregular tightenings would suggest the possibility of a UTI. Whilst the urinalysis findings are inconclusive, a formal urine culture should be undertaken. However, one should remain vigilant to the possibility of superimposed pre-eclampsia, and any increase in the degree of proteinuria should be formally quantified.

(A70) C. This patient demonstrates a white-coat effect on her blood pressure; however, the more relevant item in the scenario is the fact that she had a positive GTT. A fetal growth scan is therefore indicated to monitor for the development of macrosomia and polyhydramnios.

Q15

(A71) N. This woman's labour should be augmented to avoid prolonged labour and the development of chorioamnionitis.

(A72) J. This patient with sickle cell disease has evidence of a UTI on urinalysis. The initial measure would be the administration of intravenous antibiotics and rehydration to avert a sickle crisis.

(A73) C. The result of the FBC taken immediately after delivery is likely to be an overestimate of the actual Hb concentration, as haemodilution would not have taken place yet. This patient has a pre-existing anaemia and is unlikely to be tolerant of blood loss.

(A74) H. As this patient has not attended antenatal care for some time, her Hb was not rechecked and she has not received any treatment. It is therefore advisable to establish whether significant anaemia is present, as this may have an impact on her management in terms of precautions in the third stage or in the event of operative delivery.

(A75) G. Fetal blood sampling is contraindicated, as it could result in significant fetal bleeding in cases of fetal thrombocytopaenia. In the presence of a pathological CTG before full dilatation, Caesarean section is the only reasonable option.

Q16

These questions are based on the RCOG Green Top Guideline on the Investigation and Management of the Small-For-Gestational-Age Fetus. (See also www.rcog.org.uk/resources/Public/pdf/Small_Gest_Age_Fetus_No31.pdf.)

(A76) E. Absent or reversed end-diastolic flow in the umbilical artery after 34 weeks' gestation should prompt delivery, as the benefit of gaining maturity by temporising is substantially smaller than before 34 weeks. This is particularly relevant here as the patient presented with reduced fetal movements.

(A77) J. In this particular case scenario, extreme prematurity is combined with severe fetal growth restriction; the prospect of intact survival is negligible. Venous Dopplers play an important role as they may assist temporising in order to gain maturity; normal venous Dopplers would suggest that further watchful waiting should be considered.

(A78) B. In the presence of asymmetrical growth restriction and oligohydramnios near term, delivery should be considered. There is no contraindication to vaginal delivery, and particularly in a parous woman induction of labour can be attempted. However it should be made clear to the patient that there is a substantial risk of Caesarean section in the process.

(A79) H. This fetus should be karyotyped, as significant growth restriction with a normal or increased amount of amniotic fluid carries a high risk of fetal abnormality. In the presence of polyhydramnios, where the estimated fetal weight is below the 3rd centile for gestation, the risk of aneuploidy or a congenital malformation is at least 40%.

(A80) G. Fetal heart rate monitoring is indicated in the presence of absent or reversed end-diastolic flow, essentially screening for unprovoked decelerations. Additionally, biophysical profile and twice-weekly umbilical and middle cerebral artery Doppler should be included in the surveillance programme.

Intrapartum care

Q17

(A81) J. This is a situation where a mid-cavity forceps delivery is appropriate. The Pajot manoeuvre, which is essentially the application of vertical pressure on the shanks of the forceps, will aid the correct direction of traction during the delivery.

(A82) H. The sacroposterior position at this stage is clearly unfavourable because it results in an occipitoposterior position of the fetal head, with all its disadvantages. Once the head is in the pelvis, rotating the baby is very difficult and can lead to spinal injury if performed without disengagement of the head – it should therefore be avoided. The most appropriate manoeuvre to perform in this situation is the Prague manoeuvre, which aids flexion of the head.

(A83) B. According to the case scenario, McRoberts manoeuvre and suprapubic pressure have already been employed. The next step will involve either a rotational manoeuvre such as Rubin's, or the extraction of the posterior arm.

(A84) F. The most important rule of the singleton breech delivery is DO NOT PULL. The breech second twin is likely to be less problematic than a singleton breech, however where an assisted breech delivery of the second twin is being performed (as opposed to breech extraction), it is reasonable to adhere to the same rule. However, once the baby has delivered to the level of the inferior scapular angle, a more proactive approach may be taken. The next step would be delivery of the arms by Lövset's manoeuvre.

(A85) **A.** This is a favourable position. You have a choice of Moriceau-Smellie-Veit or Burns-Marshall manoeuvre; alternatively, a forceps can be applied to the aftercoming head. The Bracht manoeuvre, favoured in some countries, is not commonly performed in the UK because of the uncontrolled delivery of the head.

Q18

(A86) **D.** This patient presents in advanced labour with a fetus that is presenting by the breech. No information is provided on the station of the presenting part, however the likelihood of successful vaginal delivery in this patient is very high. The candidate should remember that the evidence from the Canadian Term Breech Trial cannot be simply extrapolated to preterm delivery, or to women presenting in advanced labour. In this case the fetus should be monitored continuously, as fetal compromise – as well as delay in the second stage – would necessitate delivery by Caesarean section.

(A87) **D.** There is no contraindication to vaginal delivery. The deceleration which was heard on auscultation was synchronous with the contraction, i.e. early; additionally, a single deceleration as described cannot form the basis for a management plan. What is required in this case is continuous fetal monitoring because of prematurity and maternal diabetes, but also to enable a more comprehensive assessment of the fetal heart rate pattern.

(A88) **A.** Although the first stage was prolonged, there is no indication for immediate operative delivery. An FBS is indicated because of a pathological CTG.

(A89) **L.** This patient has been in the second stage for almost two hours, with one hour of active maternal effort. The presenting part is at the level of the ischial spines, but there is no evidence of obstructed labour and a vaginal delivery is not contraindicated. The patient will require a rotational delivery and ventouse is the instrument of choice, with the correct choice of cup. Because of this patient's high parity, some clinical doubt has to remain as to why spontaneous delivery has not occurred, and the procedure should be performed in theatre in readiness for Caesarean section, i.e. as a trial of instrumental delivery. Variable decelerations with normal baseline variability would classify the CTG as suspicious rather than pathological, so that conservative measures, such as change of position or correction of hypotension, would be adopted. The depth of the deceleration is immaterial – during variable decelerations the heart rate often drops significantly. So long as the decelerations are not atypical, or associated with other adverse features, conservative measures are a good initial approach. As we are aiming to deliver this patient, we will be resolving this issue proactively.

(A90) F. In light of the low viral load, vaginal delivery is not contraindicated. Furthermore, emergency Caesarean section in labour does not appear to have the same protective effect as elective Caesarean delivery. However, as this patient's membranes have ruptured at an unknown point in time and her contractions are irregular, labour should be augmented to expedite delivery. Caesarean section should be performed if progress is suboptimal to avoid prolonged labour. Intravenous zidovudine should be administered on admission, and continued until the clamping of the umbilical cord.

Q19

(A91) B. The best approach in this case could be debated, and the choice of the mode of delivery in this patient requires good judgement. However, she appears to have made good progress in labour, the baby is appropriately grown for 34 weeks' gestation, the presentation and position are favourable, and the presenting part is below the level of the ischial spines. Instrumental delivery with the presenting part at a station higher than ischial spines +2 but with a fully engaged head is classified as mid-pelvic delivery; a station at ischial spines +2 or below is a low pelvic operation. Outlet delivery requires the presenting part to be at or on the perineum. Fetal indications for operative vaginal delivery include prolapse of the umbilical cord, premature separation of the placenta and a non-reassuring fetal heart rate. Prematurity below 34 weeks is an argument against the use of ventouse, but there is insufficient evidence to establish the safety of ventouse between 34–36 weeks. Overall, this patient is a candidate for forceps delivery, which carries a smaller maternal risk than emergency Caesarean section.

(A92) E. There is no indication for intervention at this point beyond encouraging maternal effort. Prolonged second stage of labour is defined as more than three hours with and more than two hours without regional analgesia in the nulliparous woman. In multiparous women the corresponding time intervals are two and one hour respectively.

(A93) B. Low forceps delivery is indicated here because of prolonged second stage of labour. The best estimate is of three hours in the second stage. The station of the presenting part is now at the level of ischial spines +2 and the position is occipitoanterior. Ventouse is probably better avoided because of the possibility of prematurity. A forceps delivery is the best option.

(A94) F. This woman has been in the second stage of labour for three hours, whilst the expected duration in a multipara without an epidural block is 60 minutes. Uterine contractions are infrequent at 2/10, but the history of the labour cautions against the use of oxytocin. Ventouse or forceps should not be performed where the presenting part is above the ischial spines.

(A95) **A.** In any clinical situation where the fetus may be at an increased risk of haemorrhage, fetal blood sampling and vacuum extraction (as well as difficult rotational delivery) should be avoided. In this scenario, the presenting part is at the level of the ischial spines +1 and the head is engaged and in a DOA position. As the patient's labour progressed at a reasonable rate and the head is fully engaged, provided there are no signs of obstruction such as irreducible moulding, a forceps delivery is a reasonable option. However, if any clinical doubt exists the patient should be delivered by Caesarean section.

Q20

Before tackling these questions the candidates are advised to read the RCOG Green Top Guideline on Shoulder Dystocia. (See also www.rcog.org.uk/resources/Public/pdf/shoulder_dystocia_42.pdf.)

(A96) **B.** This patient should be offered the option of elective Caesarean delivery. Apart from her BMI, there were no other risk factors for shoulder dystocia in her last pregnancy, such as postmaturity, induction of labour or macrosomia. Additionally, her previous child has sustained lasting disabilities in the process.

(A97) **A.** In the absence of macrosomia or polyhydramnios there is no indication for induction of labour. The patient has well-controlled GDM; she does not require insulin therapy, but manages with diet alone – a routine induction of labour at term is therefore not required.

(A98) **A.** There is no evidence to support induction of labour in women who have a large-for-dates fetus in the absence of diabetes mellitus. Induction of labour leads to increase in intervention without improvement in outcome.

(A99) **B.** Induction of labour in women with diabetes and fetal macrosomia does not reduce the morbidity of shoulder dystocia; if there is concern about the fetal size in a diabetic pregnancy, consideration should be given to delivery by Caesarean section.

(A100) **A.** The likely contributing factor to the shoulder dystocia in the patient's first pregnancy was the rotational instrumental delivery. The fact that she had a normal uncomplicated delivery of a 4600 g baby subsequently suggests that the risk of subsequent shoulder dystocia is not significantly higher than background risk, although the situation would need to be reviewed if rotational instrumental delivery was again required – a Caesarean section may be considered the safer alternative.

General gynaecology

Q21

(A101) B. Both the case history and histology suggest atrophic endometrium.

(A102) M. The history of erratic cycles as well as the poorly developed glands in the endometrial sample support a histological diagnosis of dyssynchronous endometrium.

(A103) E. This patient has an ectopic pregnancy; the histology describes the Arias-Stella reaction in decidualised endometrium.

(A104) C. The clinical scenario describes a woman with luteal phase deficiency.

(A105) L. Women with PCOS are at risk of developing endometrial hyperplasia because of unopposed oestrogen stimulation resulting from anovulatory cycles.

Q22

(A106) C. This is a parous woman who is trying for a pregnancy, who is also presenting with heavy painful periods. Clinical examination and pelvic ultrasound are consistent with small fibroids. The cause of her secondary infertility is unclear from the history given. Given the drop in her haemoglobin, treatment with tranexamic acid seems the best option whilst further investigations for infertility are carried out.

(A107) I. This is a nulliparous woman with heavy periods, who presents after failed initial medical treatment by her GP. Hysteroscopic removal of the fibroid may relieve her menorrhagia and may also improve her chances of fertility. Removal of submucous fibroids can be done using laser or a resectoscope. Fibroids that are totally within the cavity (grade 0) are easier to remove than those with more than 50% inside the cavity (grade 1), whilst fibroids with less than 50% inside the cavity (grade 2) may require multiple attempts for successful removal.

(A108) J. Hysterectomy with conservation of the ovaries appears to be a good option for this patient. However, her high BMI and previous Caesarean sections increase the risks associated with surgery. Endometrial ablation is contraindicated with a history of three prior Caesarean sections, as the risk of thermal injury to surrounding organs increases. There is some evidence that Mirena® IUS may be effective in a fibroid uterus, but there is a higher incidence of irregular bleeding and expulsion. On balance, the Mirena® IUS may be an option to be considered first.

(A109) C. The management of this patient poses a number of difficulties. Hysterectomy or endometrial ablation is contraindicated as she wishes to conceive. Whilst other causes of infertility have not been ruled out, the presence of fibroids may be a contributing factor and can also cause miscarriage. There are reported cases of pregnancy after uterine artery embolisation but the incidence is low, and caution should be exercised in patients wanting a pregnancy. On the other hand, her history suggests the need for great caution if a myomectomy is contemplated. Tranexamic acid seems to be the best solution whilst further investigations and counselling is undertaken with regards to her prospect of pregnancy.

(A110) D. Expectant management is indicated in this patient. Removal of a cervical fibroid could be difficult and is associated with a substantial risk of bleeding requiring a hysterectomy. Her periods have not resumed and there is no indication that they have been problematic in the past. There is a need for further investigations and surveillance with regards to the fibroid location, growth and renal function.

Q23

(A111) L. This woman is experiencing worsening pelvic pain and analgesics have failed to control her symptoms. Further empirical treatment is unlikely to be successful and the symptoms warrant a diagnostic laparoscopy to rule out endometriosis or old PID.

(A112) H. This woman had laparoscopic sterilisation two years ago; it could therefore be reasonably expected that pelvic pathology would have been seen and noted at the time of the procedure. The pain does not interfere with normal activity, and clinical examination is normal. It is unlikely that she has significant pathology, and reassurance and observation seem appropriate.

(A113) I. The symptoms and clinical examination suggest irritable bowel syndrome, and it would be appropriate to prescribe mebeverine and assess whether that resolves her symptoms before proceeding further. Mebeverine is a direct-acting smooth muscle relaxant that has relatively few adverse effects.

(A114) M. The symptoms are suggestive of subacute intestinal obstruction; this will require adhesiolysis. Laparoscopy is contraindicated in this case.

(A115) **G.** This patient has cyclical pelvic pain, the exact cause of which is uncertain. Possible causes include endometriosis or old PID. There is a place here for conservative management in the first instance. Mefenamic acid may provide symptomatic relief, although full STD screening should be undertaken and treatment administered if required.

Q24

(A116) **B.** The history is suggestive of endometriosis; although she had an emergency laparoscopy five years previously, the disease may not have been present at the time – she was on the COCP at the time of her previous laparoscopy.

(A117) **A.** IVF is likely to be the best option for this patient, however her endometriosis will require treatment first. Laparoscopic cystectomy for ovarian endometrioma is better than drainage and coagulation, and is recommended for endometriomas ≥4 cm in diameter. Excisional surgery reduces recurrence and improves spontaneous pregnancy rates in subfertile women. Laparoscopic ovarian cystectomy is recommended for ovarian endometriomas ≥4 cm as it also improves access to follicles, and possibly improves ovarian response during IVF.

(A118) **L.** TAH and BSO is the definitive treatment for this patient, whose symptoms remain disabling despite conservative management. Her family is complete, and her age and long use of contraception suggest a low risk of regret.

(A119) **J.** Ablation of endometriotic lesions reduces endometriosis-associated pain. Patients should be counselled regarding the risk of recurrent or persistent pain, either because of incomplete excision or recurrent disease. Surgery is indicated in this case where medical treatment has not proved successful. Conservative surgery may be preferable to unilateral oophorectomy.

(A120) H. This patient has a long history of endometriosis, and further investigations are unwarranted. LNG-IUS is effective for endometriosis-associated pain, and may be appropriate for this patient, who wants to space her pregnancies. Propranolol is used for prophylaxis against migraine, which is a contraindication to the COCP but not Mirena®.

Q25

(A121) G. Uterine perforation can complicate uterine instrumentation of any kind. The risk of perforation during a hysteroscopy has been reported at 0.6–1.5%, although it occurs more commonly during operative rather than diagnostic procedures. Perforation during cervical dilatation is well described, although fundal perforation with the hysteroscope or another instrument may occur. A non-pregnant uterus is unlikely to bleed significantly following perforation; however, bowel or vascular injury may occur through inadvertent abdominal instrumentation, particularly when using thermal equipment.

(A122) G. Uterine perforation during a surgical termination of pregnancy attracts substantial morbidity. The rate of confirmed perforations in one large American series was approximately 0.9/1000, with the seniority of the operator being the most powerful predictor. There is a trend to lower injury rates with cervical preparation. Bleeding can be significant and may result in hysterectomy. A perforation during suction curettage will always require a laparotomy to inspect bowel and repair the injury.

(A123) J. A number of complications would need to be discussed with the patient prior to the procedure, including bladder injury, bleeding and infection. However, the most relevant item, given the combination of continence surgery and a regional block, is urinary retention.

(A124) **A.** Abdominal distension and nausea and vomiting are suggestive of bowel injury; in this case it is probably thermal injury. It is usually associated with uterine perforation; however, it has been described without perforation, particularly in women with myometrial defects such as previous Caesarean sections. Pyrexia and a raised WBC would be expected when peritonitis develops; this patient is presenting with symptoms of ileus which may precede peritonitis.

(A125) **D.** Laparoscopy carries a risk of intestinal injury of approximately 0.6:1000, with most incidents occurring during entry. Interestingly, whilst open entry techniques reduce the risk of vascular injury, they don't seem to have the same protective effect on bowel injury. In this patient, the site of surgery (rectovaginal septum) clearly increased the risk of bowel damage.

Q26

(A126) **A.** Lichen sclerosus can occur in any age group. Skin in the whole genital region may be affected, including the peri-anal area and genitocrural folds. The skin has well-demarcated whitening that does not extend to the vaginal mucosa. Pruritus is a common associated symptom.

(A127) **A.** The classical histological features are an atrophic epidermis with overlying hyperkeratosis, an effaced dermo-epidermal junction, superficial dermal hyalinisation and lymphocytic infiltration.

(A128) **B.** Seborrhoeic dermatitis (eczema) is a common condition. The vulva is often affected; other affected sites include the scalp and flexural areas, e.g. between the breasts, in the axilla and in vulval creases. The skin appears red, scaly and inflamed. Scratching may cause excoriation and lichenification. Histologically, there is parakeratosis, papillomatosis and spongiosis. The absence of neutrophil infiltrates in the epidermis helps differentiate the lesion from psoriasis.

(A129) E. Vulval psoriatic lesions are well defined, uniform and symmetrical. The appearance is that of a beefy-red area that may affect any part of the vulva, but not the vaginal mucosa. Characteristic lesions may be present in other locations. Histologically, there is papillomatosis, parakeratosis with neutrophil exocytosis and spongiform pustules.

(A130) F. The lesions described are likely to represent herpes simplex. The differential diagnosis of genital ulcers also includes chancroid and syphilis.

Endocrinology and infertility

Q27

(A131) I. Non-classical adult-onset adrenal hyperplasia is a differential diagnosis that can be distinguished from polycystic ovary syndrome by basal 17-hydroxyprogesterone measurement. The prevalence of non-classical CAH varies according to population from 1% to 19%. Most patients with either PCOS or non-classical CAH will have elevated DHEAS androstendione and testosterone. Basal 17-hydroxyprogesterone (17-OHP) levels <200 ng/dl (0.6 nmol/l) effectively rule out 21-OH-deficient CAH, whilst levels >500 ng/dl (15.1 nmol/l) confirm the diagnosis.

(A132) A. Patients with subclinical hypothyroidism have an elevated TSH and normal T4. Measurement of thyroid antibodies is a useful test to detect those who are likely to progress to overt disease.

(A133) G. Patients with Cushing syndrome have chronic excess of glucocorticoids. Differential diagnosis includes obesity, PCOS, diabetes mellitus and hirsutism. Cushing disease refers to the presence of an ACTH-producing pituitary adenoma. The classic syndrome includes obesity, amenorrhoea, hypertension, glucose intolerance, hirsutism, striae, muscle weakness, osteoporosis, purpura and bruising, and psychiatric disorders. A 24-hour urinary-free cortisol determination is a useful test. Also useful is late-evening plasma cortisol. Urinary 17-hydroxycorticosteroids and measurement of morning and afternoon plasma cortisol are less reliable because of the overlap between normal and abnormal. CRH stimulation test can be useful to distinguish Cushing syndrome from other causes of raised cortisol.

(A134) H. CRH stimulation test is useful in assessing the source of raised cortisol. In Cushing disease, but not in ectopic ACTH syndrome, there is elevated plasma cortisol and ACTH following intravenous administration of CRH. Also useful is the dexamethasone suppression test.

(A135) D. The history, including the use of venlafaxine (a serotonin and noradrenaline reuptake inhibitor, SNRI), should raise the possibility of hyperprolactinaemia.

Q28

(A136) H. This patient's symptoms are consistent with a pheochromocytoma. It is clear that differential diagnosis is complex; however, making the correct diagnosis is of utmost importance, as malignancy can occur in 10% of patients. There is substantial cardiovascular morbidity, including hypertension, arrhythmias and myocarditis, as well as neurological sequelae of severe hypertension. Symptoms may include palpitations, tremor, weakness, headaches, tiredness, weight loss and many others.

(A137) L. This patient's results indicate hyperprolactinaemia. Hyperprolactinaemia is the most common hypothalamo-pituitary endocrine disorder. Mildly increased levels may be physiological, however a sustained or significant increase should be investigated. Raised prolactin levels may be idiopathic, secondary to drugs such as phenothiazines (antipsychotics), or a result of a pituitary micro- or macroadenoma; it may be raised in other endocrine disorders such as hypothyroidism. Typically, it will present with oligo- or amenorrhoea, galactorrhoea or, where a tumour is the cause, with visual field defects and/or headaches. Imaging of the sella region should always be performed as part of the investigation. The follicles visualised on USS would be the result of anovulation.

(A138) **M.** The features of this case are not typical of PCOS and suggest Cushing syndrome, which needs to be excluded.

(A139) **J.** This patient has a number of features of PCOS, such as menstrual disturbance, obesity, inverse LH/FSH ratio and a positive USS. Additionally, she has impaired glucose tolerance. As her two-hour glucose value is <11.2 mmol/l, she does not have overt diabetes.

(A140) **K.** Craniopharyngioma may pose a difficult differential diagnosis with pituitary tumours. However, symptoms and signs of raised intracranial pressure and weight loss are not commonly seen with micro- or macroadenomas. Craniopharyngiomas peak in childhood and between 40 and 60 years of age. The majority (75%) are suprasellar in location.

Q29

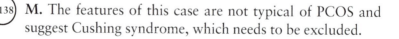

(A141) **A.** This patient with hyperprolactinaemia should undergo appropriate investigation to exclude the need for surgical therapy. Where surgical therapy is not required, cabergoline would be the appropriate choice of drug. Cabergoline is a dopamine agonist with proven efficacy in idiopathic hyperprolactinaemia, micro- and macroadenoma, and empty sella syndrome. It appears to have better efficacy than bromocriptine as well as a more favourable safety profile. The administration is weekly rather than daily.

(A142) **I.** This patient appears to be insulin resistant. The most appropriate drug would be one that improves insulin sensitivity, whilst addressing some of her other symptoms.

Metformin, which is a biguanide, would be the most appropriate drug.

(A143) F. This patient appears to have a clearly defined problem with increased hair growth in one particular, relatively small, area of her body. As there are no other symptoms to address and the affected surface area is small, a topical agent might be most appropriate. Eflornithine is the first licensed topical hair retardant in the UK. The mode of action is decreasing androgen sensitivity of hair follicles. You may wish to consider that cyproterone acetate is the only licensed *systemic* agent for the treatment of hirsutism. Interestingly (and perhaps more importantly on the more global scale of health), eflornithine, marketed as Ornidyl® rather than Vaniqua®, is effective in combating sleeping sickness.

(A144) B. This combination of anti-androgen and estrogen is used as a COCP (Dianette®).

(A145) J. This patient is actively trying for a pregnancy. The feature of oligomenorrhoea suggests anovulatory cycles. Clomid ovulation induction is therefore appropriate, although a normal semen analysis and tubal patency should be first ascertained.

Q30

(A146) B. Ovulation induction using clomiphene citrate is appropriate.

(A147) C. Absent periods for six months would usually be taken as the cut-off for diagnosis of amenorrhoea and instigation of investigations. Basic investigations in this case are normal and it would be appropriate to await events.

(A148) B. Clomiphene citrate is the first choice for women with inadequate luteal phase. The only significant risk is that of multiple pregnancy. The usual starting dose is 50 mg a day for five days, starting on days three, four or five of the cycle.

 A. Treatment with IUI improves fertility in minimal to mild endometriosis. This patient was managed expectantly for two years since she had surgical ablation for endometriosis; although IVF is a consideration, there is no tubal damage or male factor infertility, and so it would be appropriate to await the outcome of IUI.

 I. IVF should be considered here, as there is evidence of endometriosis involving tubes and ovaries. Further expectant management is not the best option given her age and the long history of infertility. One should bear in mind that endometriomas should be treated surgically to improve fertility.

Q31

E. Overall success rate of IVF in women aged 23–35 years is quoted as >20%.

C. The Odds Ratio of congenital malformations (minor and major) following IVF is reported at approximately twice the background risk. However, studies have not produced consistent results.

D. Success rate following IVF for women in this age group.

H. The reason for the wide range of success rates is the variation in method of sterilisation and the resultant residual tubal length, as well as operator experience in reversal surgery.

E. The natural conception rate in each cycle is approximately 20–25%.

Urogynaecology

Q32

(A156) **A.** The initial management of stress incontinence should include lifestyle advice (weight loss, etc.) and pelvic floor exercise.

(A157) **B.** Immediate-release non-proprietary oxybutynin should be offered to women with OAB or mixed urinary incontinence as first-line drug treatment if bladder training has been ineffective. If immediate-release oxybutynin is not well tolerated, darifenacin, solifenacin, tolterodine, trospium or an extended-release or transdermal formulation of oxybutynin should be considered as alternatives. There is no evidence of a clinically important difference in efficacy between anti-muscarinic drugs. However, immediate-release non-proprietary oxybutynin is the most cost-effective of the available options.

(A158) **H.** Moclobemide is a reversible monamino-oxidase inhibitor. Concomitant use of duloxetine is contraindicated. Many surgical procedures are available for the treatment of urinary stress incontinence. Retropubic mid-urethral tape, colposuspension and autologous rectus fascial sling have comparable effectiveness. However, retropubic mid-urethral tape procedures consume less hospital resources and are associated with faster recovery. Tension-free vaginal tape involves use of monofilament macropore polypropylene mesh.

(A159) **I.** Treatment options for OAB that does not respond to conservative treatment are limited. Antimuscarinic drugs may worsen coronary heart disease, congestive heart failure and arrhythmias. Data on the use of botulinum toxin A in the management of detrusor overactivity are limited, but show cure or improvement in about half of patients. Benefit may last between 3–12 months. Botulinum toxin B appears to be effective for a duration of about six weeks. Weighed against major surgical interventions with high morbidity, botulinum toxin A is a consideration for this patient.

(A160)   E. Duloxetine should not routinely be used as a second-line treatment for women with urinary stress incontinence; however, this patient is not an ideal candidate for surgical treatment. Her urinary symptoms may improve with weight loss.

Gynaecological oncology

Q33

(A161) B. This is stage IIb endometrial cancer, and adjuvant therapy is therefore required, usually in the form of external beam.

(A162) E. In locally invasive cancer of the cervix, chemoradiation confers a survival benefit at five years, which has been quoted at about 12%.

(A163) F. Carcinoma of the Fallopian tube behaves in a similar way to ovarian cancer, despite having the same embryological origin as the uterus. It is therefore managed by TAH and BSO, omentectomy and selective lymphadenectomy. Cancer of the Fallopian tube is chemosensitive and responds to agents used in the treatment of ovarian cancer.

(A164) F. This is a stage III ovarian cancer, requiring chemotherapy.

(A165) A. Patients with one (and possibly two) micrometastases (<5 mm) do not require adjuvant radiation therapy. Pelvic and groin irradiation is indicated in patients with macrometastases (>10 mm), patients with extracapsular spread, and patients with two (or possibly three) or more micrometastases.

Q34

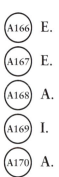 E.

A167 E.

A168 A.

A169 I.

A170 A.

Therapeutics in obstetrics and gynaecology

Q35

(A171) J. This patient has diabetes, but has no other risk factors of arterial disease. The COCP can be used with caution. A low-strength preparation containing 20 mcg ethinylestradiol would have been particularly suitable; however, she has mid-cycle bleeding, and thus a standard strength or a phased preparation is more likely to work. Biphasic and triphasic preparations contain ethinylestradiol and levonorgestrel or ethinylestradiol and norethisterone.

(A172) E. This patient's needs are more likely to be met by a depot preparation of longer duration. Etonogestrel 68 mg contained in implantable subdermal rods (Implanon®, Organon®) provides contraception for three years. Other depot preparations include medroxyprogesterone acetate (Depo-Provera®, Pharmacia), which provides protection for 12 weeks, and norethisterone enanthate (Noristerat®, Shering Health), which provides contraception for eight weeks.

(A173) F. COCP reduces milk production; this patient, despite having used the COCP successfully in the past, is a candidate for the POP. In the UK, progestogens used in oral POP are ethynodiol diacetate (Femulen®, Pharmacia), norethisterone (Micronor®, Janssen-Cilag), desogestrel (Cerazette®,

Organon®) and levonorgestrel (Microval®, Wyeth and Norgeston®, Schering Health).

(A174) F. This patient is a candidate for progestogen-only contraception. The presence of a fibroid uterus presents an added difficulty. As she is uncertain of her plans for pregnancy and given her age, long-term depot preparations may not be ideal.

(A175) D. COCP is suitable treatment for endometriosis, but is contraindicated in this patient because of a history of hypertension. Gestrinone 2.5 mg twice weekly can be used to treat endometriosis. Depot preparations may be considered as an alternative.

Q36

(A176) A. Emergency contraception containing levonorgestrel is effective if taken within 72 hours of unprotected intercourse. The longer the latency since intercourse, the lower the success rate. The effective dose is 1.5 mg as a single dose or in two divided doses 12 hours apart; it should taken as soon as possible after intercourse, and preferably within 12 hours.

(A177) D. Third-generation progestogens (desogestrel and gestodene) and drospirenone may be considered for women who have progestogenic side-effects such as acne, headache, depression, weight gain or breast discomfort on second-generation COCP. These are also effective for women with breakthrough bleeding.

(A178) G. Subdermal implants containing etonogestrel are inserted during the first five days of the cycle. The single flexible rod is inserted subdermally into the medial aspect of the upper arm and is effective for up to three years.

(A179) F. The features are suggestive of hyperandrogenism and PCOS. The antiandrogen cyproterone acetate should be considered.

(A180) H. Transdermal patches releasing norelgestromin 150 mcg/24 hours, and ethinylestradiol 20 mcg/24 hours, are suitable options for this patient. The patch is applied once weekly for three weeks followed by a patch-free week.

Q37

(A181) D. Vitamin D is the most relevant supplement in osteoporosis, often administered in conjunction with calcium.

(A182) I. Folinic acid rescue in methotrexate toxicity.

(A183) E. Folic acid supplementation periconceptually is associated with a decrease in NTDs. Women with specific risk factors should receive the higher dose, i.e. 5 mg rather than 0.4 mg.

(A184) F. Women with severe hyperemesis, particularly where associated with deranged liver function tests, are at risk of developing Wernicke's encephalopathy. This risk is reduced by thiamine administration. Usually, thiamine will have to be administered intravenously as, by definition, women at most risk are unlikely to tolerate oral therapy; it is important to monitor for anaphylaxis.

(A185) G. Women with obstetric cholestasis are at risk of postpartum haemorrhage because of a deficiency in vitamin K-dependent clotting factors. Vitamin K should therefore be supplemented orally for four weeks prior to planned – or likely – delivery.

Audit, research and management

Q38

(A186) E. Patients have a right to refuse to participate in clinical research. It is important though to examine the characteristics of those who refuse to participate, because refusal by a specific subgroup is a form of selection bias that needs to be considered by the investigators to assess its possible impact on the outcomes of the study and the generalisability of its conclusions.

(A187) E. Because only a subset of smears was re-examined, there is a possibility of selection bias. Given how the study was conducted, the stated conclusion cannot be drawn. A random sample selected from all smears examined by the laboratory could have avoided this problem.

(A188) G. Assessment bias is the form of bias that blind and double-blind trials are designed to overcome. In this study, the response of subjects and the assessments made by the researchers may have been influenced by their knowledge of the type of treatment received during the study. However, blinding in trials involving surgery is difficult unless sham procedures and placebo are used, and this raises ethical questions which may be difficult to overcome, resulting in trials failing to receive approval from ethics committees.

(A189) C. Screening bias is a type of selection bias which occurs in screening programmes; those who comply with a screening programme tend to be generally healthier and at a lower risk compared to non-participants. There are a number of reasons for this, including socio-demographic factors. There is a risk that the better outcome noted in participants be wrongly attributed to the screening programme. Length, or length-time, bias occurs in diseases which present across a broad spectrum of biologic activity; some patients have aggressive, rapidly growing tumours with a short asymptomatic phase, whilst others have less aggressive tumours with longer latency and an inherently better prognosis. These less aggressive tumours will be more likely to be identified in a screening programme, and, even without therapy, the cohort identified by screening will have a better prognosis. Lead-time bias occurs when the disease has a long asymptomatic period which is not taken into account. Here, it is possible that screening may result in early diagnosis, but the natural history remains unaltered, for example because of the absence of effective intervention.

(A190) D. Studies based on recall of past events will be subject to recall bias. In such cases, corroborating evidence from other sources, e.g. hospital or general practice case-notes, could be helpful.

Q39

(A191) N. The hazard ratio gives the observed event rate in the study group as a proportion of the expected occurrence of the event.

(A192) H. The Chi-squared (χ^2) test is used to compare the distribution of categorical variables in two samples. The Chi-squared (χ^2) test is carried out on the *actual numbers* of occurrences, not on percentages, proportions or means of observations. The null hypothesis is that there is no association between the two variables.

(A193)   C. The unpaired (independent variables) t-test is used to compare two sets of quantitative data where samples are collected independently of one another. It tests the null hypothesis that the population means related to two independent, random samples from an approximately normal distribution are equal.

(A194)   G. The general purpose of multiple regression analysis is to examine the relationship between several independent or predictor variables and a dependent variable.

(A195)   M. The Kaplan-Meier survival curve provides an estimate of the survival function from life-time data, such as the fraction of patients who remain disease free over time following surgery. A Kaplan-Meier survival curve consists of a series of horizontal steps of declining magnitude which depict the true survival function. In the given scenario the curve could estimate the proportion of women over time who continue to consider their treatment successful.

Q40

(A196)   A. Although radiotherapy and radical surgery have different consequences beyond survival, these were not considered. The analysis was restricted to a single natural unit (post-treatment survival), and no attempt is made to value the output.

(A197)   I. When comparing two programmes that differ in no significant respect and accomplish the outcome of interest, the comparison becomes essentially a search for the least-cost alternative. This type of comparison is a cost-minimisation analysis.

(A198)   A. This analysis compares diagnostic strategies in terms of cost per case detected. Typically, cost-effectiveness analysis considers a single measure of output measured in the most appropriate units, and no attempt is made to value the output.

(A199) F. Cost-benefit analysis attempts to value the consequences of interventions in monetary terms. The difficulties encountered in valuing outcomes in monetary terms often mean that this type of analysis becomes restricted to measurable outcomes. Willingness to pay is one technique used to assess outcomes, where patients are asked to put a monetary value on particular aspects of the service (e.g. easy parking at the hospital, clinic running on time, etc).

(A200) C. This type of analysis is used when outcomes are not identical. In this scenario the outcome of hysterectomy is amenorrhoea, whilst ablation may also result in reduced menstrual flow as well as a number of failures and possibly reoperation over years of follow-up. Thus, cost-utility analysis is used to compare single or multiple effects that are not necessarily common to both arms. The analysis is achieved when the outputs are adjusted according to preference or utility scores. In other words, the comparison becomes that of the quality of (for example) life-years gained, not simply the number of years.

Ethics and law in obstetrics and gynaecology

Whilst working on the following questions, the candidates should take into consideration that it would be unusual for only one ethical or medico-legal principle to apply in any case, and the relative importance of each is a matter that requires some judgement. In the following questions on ethics and medical law, we give the candidates the opportunity to work on determining the overriding or most applicable principle in each case.

Q41

(A201) I. The patient's autonomy necessitates that she consents to interventions on her person which, during pregnancy, includes any interventions on behalf of the fetus. However, at birth the fetus becomes a person with rights, and the mother's autonomy cannot override actions judged to be in the best interest of the baby.

(A202) J. Erb's palsy is a known complication of shoulder dystocia. The occurrence of a complication is not in itself proof of negligence. Judgement on the conduct of delivery will rest on the opinion of the court with reference to the Bolam test. The Bolam test is based on the ruling of a trial judge in the Bolam case in 1957. He said: 'A doctor is not guilty of negligence if he has acted in accordance with a practice accepted as proper by a responsible body of medical opinion skilled in that particular art, even though a body of adverse opinion also exists amongst medical men.' In essence this puts peer judgement at the centre of assessing clinical care.

(A203) G. It is unlikely that a scenario exists where a single ethical principle applies to the exclusion of others. However, adherence to the truth is a binding obligation on doctors and takes a central place within the ethical framework of the patient–doctor relationship. Disclosure of errors in test results can be distressing to a number of patients, whether or not they consequently received unnecessary or inadequate treatment. In all cases the situation must be handled sensitively, but veracity ought to be the guiding principle.

(A204) H. Learning disability in itself is not synonymous with lack of mental capacity, and the majority of individuals with learning disabilities will be considered capable of making their own choices about their healthcare. The patient's express wishes ought not to be overridden based on the authorisation of her carers, as this could constitute battery. Under some circumstances, patients who cannot make their own choice can be treated according to doctors' judgement of what is in their best interest (here the principle of beneficence would apply).

(A205) I. This scenario should raise concern for the patient's best interest. Her husband seems to exclude the patient from decision making. Her apparent compliance may not be an expression of autonomy but simply submitting to her husband's wishes; her poor command of English and young age also make her vulnerable. Whilst cultural differences in customs and behaviour should be taken into account, they should not be allowed to infringe on the basic framework of the patient–doctor relationship.

Q42

 J. The National Health Service (Primary Care) Act 1997 requires that a doctor shall render to his patients all necessary and appropriate personal medical services of the type usually provided by general medical practitioners.

 C. The European Convention on Human Rights, Article 8 concerns the right to respect for private life, and Article 9 concerns the right to freedom of thought, conscience and religion. Both articles are taken to support the right to autonomous decision making.

A208 **C.** This patient's right to choose is enforced in the European Convention on Human Rights, Article 8 and Article 9.

A209 **G.** The Abortion Act 1967 regulates the legal framework for the provision of the service.

A210 **B.** The Human Tissue Act 2004 regulates the use of human tissue in research and audit. It repeals and replaces the Human Tissue Act 1961, the Anatomy Act 1984 and the Human Organ Transplants Act 1989 as they relate to England and Wales. The Act makes it lawful for relevant material, which has been obtained from a living person, to be stored and used for purposes considered intrinsic to the proper conduct of a patient's treatment, such as clinical audit, quality assurance and performance assessment, or those that are necessary for public health.

Index